WHY MUSIC CONDUCTORS LIVE INTO THEIR 90'S?

The Simple, Revolutionary Discovery that Can Make You Live Longer, Increase Your Stamina & Stretch, and Normalize Your Blood Pressure In Minutes

WHY DO MUSIC CONDUCTORS LIVE INTO THEIR 90'S?

The Simple Revolutionary Discovery That Can Make You Live Longer, Increase Your Stamina, & Stretch, And Normalize Your Blood Pressure In Minutes

By Prof. Steven Rochlitz

© Copyright 1993 by Steven Rochlitz
Published by Human Ecology Balancing Sciences, Inc.
P.O. Box 737, Mahopac, N.Y. 10541 USA
ISBN: 0-945262-42-6   Library of Congress Catalog Card Number: 93-33432
First printing: May, 1994   Printed in the USA
9 8 7 6 5 4 3 2 1

NOTE: The following Rochlitz creations are also trademarked: Heart Integration,™ Meridian Integration,™ Meta-Integration.™

Warning-Disclaimer

This book is designed to provide accurate, research information in regard to the subject matter covered. It is not intended to offer medical, psychological or other professional services. For medical and psychological diagnosing, prescribing and treatment, consult a licensed professional. The author and publisher shall have neither liability nor responsibility to any person or entity with respect to any alleged loss or damage alleged to be caused directly or indirectly by the information contained in this book.

Library of Congress Cataloging-in-Publication Data
Rochlitz, Steven
   Why do music conductors live into their 90'S? : the simple, revolutionary discovery that can make you live longer, increase your stamina & stretch, and normalize your blood pressure in minutes / Steven Rochlitz ; foreword by John Wright illustrations by Ken Vatter.
       p. cm.
   Includes bibliographical references and index.
   ISBN 0-945262-42-6 : $12.95
   1. Applied kinesiology. 2. Health. 3. Physical fitness.
   4. Conducting- -Health aspects.   I. Title.
   RZ251.A65R63   1993
   613.7'0446—dc20   93-33432

WHY DO MUSIC CONDUCTORS LIVE INTO THEIR 90'S?

The Simple, Revolutionary Discovery that Can Make You Live Longer, Increase Your Stamina & Stretch, and Normalize Your Blood Pressure In Minutes

By Prof. STEVEN ROCHLITZ

Foreword by John Wright, M.D.

Cover Design by Barbara Dunn
Illustrations by Ken Vatter

HUMAN ECOLOGY BALANCING SCIENCES, INC.
PUBLISHING THAT UNITES SCIENCE & HEALING

NEW YORK

To
Kitty Kopey

With
Love, Always

For it is not likely that one could meet
a person with a more...
lovely heart!

TABLE OF CONTENTS

ACKNOWLEDGEMENTS

I would like to thank the following people for their research or their communications to me: Sheldon Deal, D.C., George Goodheart, D.C., and Fred Shull, M.D.

I thank my attorney, William Unroch for his suggestions. For their support of the Human Ecology Balancing Sciences programs in the last year, I thank Ron Jahner, Dean Stonier, Libby Gardon (of Canada's Consumer Health Organization), and John O'Neill, A.P.

For their assistance on this book, I would like to thank the following people: Gal Drimmer, and Bud Colucci for their help with artwork; Barbara Dodd for the cover; Irene Yaychuk, PhD, and Kitty Kopey for proofreading. I am indebted to Roberta Johnson for editing the manuscript. Finally, for her tireless, public relations efforts, I especially thank Gloria Vivo.

FOREWORD

I suppose that everyone has a turning point in their career when some startling change takes place which inspires and stimulates a new wave of thought and a different exciting change of direction. This important moment occurred for me in November 1985 when I attended a seminar given by Prof. Steven Rochlitz in Melbourne, Australia. This seminar contained the breakthroughs in this book.

At that time of my 12 year medical career in General Practice, I was puzzled and frustrated by some of the inadequacies of my conventional, medical teaching in dealing with a significant number of patients. Those who supposedly had nothing wrong with them for all tests were normal yet they were not well and the patient knew it. And then there were those who had been told they will never be cured and that they must take drug therapy for the rest of their lives.

How exciting then to be taught a new technique that could demonstrate that their bodies were totally out of balance and therefore they were sick. By following the technique of Steven Rochlitz in balancing the body, the patient's system is readjusted so that it can start to function normally again and so give it the ability to help cure itself.

After performing these Rochlitz techniques, and if a good diet is maintained and medication is kept to the absolute minimum (or in most cases stopped), the results are quite stunning. In my practice, I have been able to achieve some notable successes and even cures. Some patients have *ceased all anti-hypertensive therapy and remained normotensive, have ceased diuretics and remained well,* have ceased antidepressants, hypnotics, sedatives and remained happy, others have overcome food allergies, irritable bowel symptoms, arthritis, vertigo, learning disorders, fatigue and eczema. They have regrown hair, regained concentration, have regained normal menstrual cycles, have lost weight, have performed better at sports and most regained energy, happiness and vitality. The methods in this book will not cure all illness and they are not the total panacea for problems but without them the body will not have a chance to heal itself.

With this book, the reader will now be able to overcome all the complaints I have outlined above. As for my medical colleagues, I hope in time the profession will accept Rochlitz' methods and that they can be taught to all keen and enthusiastic medical students. In this way, many costs of drug therapy can be saved, many patients will feel better and remain well, and the doctor will be able to treat the illness and prevent its reoccurrence rather than treat and retreat. Thank you Steve for your inspired work.

John Wright, M.D.

PREFACE

Why *do* so many music conductors live into their 90's? This book is the first to correctly answer this crucial question. Yes, the answer should allow all of us to join them in this quest for longevity — *if* we just follow the simple and safe methods of this book. You will be astounded to find out that literally *in seconds or minutes*, you can supercharge your heart and circulatory system! You will shortly partake in an historic journey! With the discoveries in this book, mankind can now learn how to attain a *vibrant* four score and ten years of life — just as many music conductors have!

Chapter one will tell you how a physicist was *forced* by life-long, ill health to make this great, medical discovery. Chapters two and three will focus on the special exercises we have devised, based on our breakthroughs in understanding music conductors' longevities. Indeed, the third chapter will reveal one special exercise which should prove to be even more beneficial than that which the conductors perform! So maybe we can even live into our proverbial 120's.

Next we will reveal diet and nutrition discoveries that can boost our chances for a very long *and* healthy life. We will learn how to significantly decrease our chances of developing cardiovascular disease and cancer. A chapter on the author's unique breakthroughs in weight loss science follows to insure our success in attaining health and longevity.

Then — what we have done to boost your heart and circulation — we will do for your brain! A similar, simple, safe and effective type of exercise can increase your reading, learning and memory capacities very rapidly.

In three additional chapters, we will zero in on the use of this book's revolutionary methods to normalize blood pressure, and to help those who suffer from chronic fatigue or Multiple Sclerosis.

We will also show you how to greatly boost your athletic abilities. Whether you are an Olympic Gold medal winner or a weekend warrior, we promise you will increase your stretch, stamina and athletic performance very rapidly!

The epilogue contains actual feedback from people who have used the breakthroughs in this book during the last few years. These people have normalized their blood pressures, eliminated their cardiac arrhythmias, safely gotten off medications, eliminated bruising, and cold hands and feet and other problems. You can send us *your* results for a future edition. Years or decades from now, you can tell us what this book has done for your longevity!

The first appendix will reveal the actual causes of today's chronic health problems. The next appendix will show you how to master the new science of Applied Kinesiology — discovered by today's best physicians. This way you can immediately find out how your body may be imbalanced and what to do about it. The remaining appendices contain helpful resources, a bibliography and an index. Footnotes, throughout the book, are referenced sequentially in the bibliography — Appendix D.

We beseech the reader — unless medically advised against — to *perform* the methods in this book *as you read them.* They are things that need to be *done — not just read —* if you want to attain the goals of longevity and health.

The methods described in this book are safe, easy, rapid, inexpensive, effective, and fun to do. The reader is invited to join the many thousands, around the world, that have either gotten well with these methods, or are using them to live into their 90's and beyond!

Prof. Steven Rochlitz
October, 1993
New York

1

A PHYSICIST DISCOVERS A MEDICAL BREAKTHROUGH

It's a well known fact that many music conductors have lived to about 90 or more. Leopold Stowkoski was 95, Pablo Casals was 96, David Mannes was 93, Paul Paray was 92, Nadia Boulanger was 90, Arturo Toscani was 89, as was Pierre Monteux, when they passed on. Even Charlie Chaplin — a comedic actor, director and producer — intrinsically knew this secret. He used it to live to 88! This is even more astounding because these people were born at a time when the average life expectancy was only about 50! Just as important as longevity is the quality of life. Music conductors are also known to be *vital* and *vibrant* throughout their lives.

Until now, no one has been able to explain why. The answer would help us all attain that most lofty of goals — a very long, and healthy life! Our logic here is simple. The average life expectancy now in civilized societies is about 75 years. The three major causes of death are heart attacks, cancer and strokes. If we can ascertain and duplicate what music conductors are doing for their hearts and cardiovascular systems we can greatly diminish the risks of heart attacks and stroke — the first and third leading causes of death, respectively. If we adhere to certain diet and nutritional recommendations made in this book, we can greatly diminish the likelihood of suffering from the second, leading cause of death — cancer. That's how we can expect to make it into our 90's. The breakthroughs in this book just might get us there and in a healthy state throughout our lives!

What has enabled this author to be the first to make the breakthroughs that may enable us to live into our 90's and beyond? We could sum it up by saying that two factors were essential. First was my education as a physicist. The second, crucial factor was that my own life-long, ill health and lack of improvement after so many visits to mainstream, medical physicians forced me to develop a truly open mind. I had many chronic, health problems from the time I was a small child. These included fatigue, gastrointestinal disorders, headaches including migraines, arthritis and more.

By the time I was 25, I had already taught physics at two Universities for two years. At that time, even my heart became affected. I began to experience various types of cardiac arrhythmias. As a scientist, I was astounded (and often disgusted) to see that the medical doctors I went to had no interest in finding the cause of my complaints! It was just take this or that drug. My scientific training, of course, told me that this was *not* science, as science deals with *cause and effect* — not merely with masking symptoms with toxic, or potentially toxic, substances that are foreign to the body.

So I knew there had to be a better and *more scientific* way. Indeed, I had no choice as I steadily worsened. I ended up near death and in a disabled state for a few years. But I had begun to study various aspects of what is called alternative, or complimentary, or holistic medicine. First I studied nutrition. This was to prove to be a double-edged sword. Just as I was to later understand that many of my symptoms came from (hidden) food allergies, allergy to some of the vitamins also occurred! Then I began to study the new medical discipline known as clinical ecology or environmental medicine. This discipline reveals that food, chemical and other environmental allergies often cause many of today's chronic, degenerative, immunological and even "psychological" illnesses. I found out from these physicians that I had "Universal allergies." This knowledge was able to prevent me from getting worse. But I was still desperately searching for wellness.

I then learned of a remarkable, new science called Applied

Kinesiology. This is the quickest way to determine imbalance in the body and to correct it. The imbalance relates to dysfunction in the nervous system or the acupuncture meridian system or to other systems. By 1983, I had used this new science to get well for the first time in my life. I then made discoveries in this new field. In 1985, I made the breakthrough — revealed in this book — that alleviated my cardiac arrhythmias, normalized my blood pressure and eliminated the chronic fatigue. My stamina and stretch were also immediately increased with this discovery of how to supercharge the heart and the circulatory system, literally in seconds or minutes. The wisdom of the body and how *quickly* it will recover — *if you just do the right thing* — never cease to amaze me.

In 1986, a physician sent me a study that showed that "arm jogging" was more beneficial for longevity than was traditional (leg) jogging. I realized *then* that my discovery in 1985 was also the answer to the marvelous riddle of why so many music conductors live into their 90's! This explanation will form the crux of this book and can lead to the possibility of *your* living into your 90's and beyond! The discoveries in this book have also led to the improvement of many cardiovascular complaints or conditions including normalizing blood pressure, and helping sufferers of Multiple Sclerosis and chronic fatigue.

Since 1985, we have also worked with all types of leading (and Sunday) athletes. They were amazed at the rapid gains in stamina, stretch and performance! Other circulation-related problems that can now be helped include bruising, cardiac arrhythmias, frozen muscles or joints, and varicose veins. We have taught these methods to people for eight years with tremendous results and virtually no side-effects.

It's your turn now to learn how to significantly increase your chances for a long and healthy life.

2

MUSIC CONDUCTORS'
LONGEVITY REVEALED:
THE ROCHLITZ HEART
INTEGRATION™
EXERCISES

In 1985, this author made a discovery[1] that history may record as a true breakthrough in mankind's age-old quest for longevity and health. It may, at last, explain why so many music conductors have lived into their 90's. In just a few pages, you will be able to *duplicate* the factor responsible for music conductors' longevities! You will shortly learn how to supercharge your heart and cardiovascular system in minutes.

But first we need to look at our current understanding of the heart. The heart has hemispheres with *differing* functions, as does the brain. One heart hemisphere sends out poorly oxygenated blood to the lungs; the other receives oxygenated blood and sends it out to the rest of the body. Many mysteries remain in our understanding of the circulatory system. The beating of the heart's four chambers and the peripheral pulses often are not at the same frequency. Russian scientists consider the heart to be a "second brain" with holographic qualities. Western researchers have recently discovered that the heart is an endocrine gland,[2] producing hormones that regulate blood pressure and interact with the other organs including the kidneys and the brain.[3] *It is far more than a simple pump.* (This chapter may indicate why mechanical hearts may never work properly.) We all know that allegory has it that thoughts and feelings are "in the heart."

Others, before us, have attempted to answer the great question of why so many music conductors live into their 90's *and* with vitality throughout their lives. Some have speculated that the classical music, conductors listen to, is the key. If this were true, *all* musicians — indeed everyone who listens to classical music — would demonstrate the longevity that conductors have. They do not. We were aware that some studies showed that exercising with the arms may be *better* (cardiovascularly) than the usual running or walking exercises. This "arm jogging" is clearly performed by music conductors, many of whom live into their 90's. Is it the particular motion that music conductors do, with their arms, every day, that has enabled so many of them to live into their 90's? *IS THIS THE SECRET? Or is it the music AND the arm motion... AND SOMETHING ELSE?*

The answers were found, by this author, through his knowledge of applied kinesiology, acupuncture theory and integration (or cross-crawl) exercises. Applied Kinesiology, a new science, was created in the 1960's by Dr. George Goodheart. It was based on his knowledge of acupuncture and muscle kinesiology. Applied kinesiology has revealed that a particular muscle is energetically connected to a corresponding, acupuncture meridian. Now, for thousands of years, the acupuncture meridians have been proven to energize their corresponding organs. (For example, the Liver meridian energizes the liver itself.) So there is an intertwined muscle/acupuncture meridian/organ connection.

Other researchers, starting with Drs. Doman and Delacato, over 40 years ago, found a certain type of exercise called "cross-crawl" was very beneficial for those who had dyslexia, or suffered an injury leading to paralysis or a disease such as Mulitple Sclerosis. Cross-crawl involves a simultaneous use of the *opposite* arm and leg. Both pairs of opposite arm and leg are used in succession. (Just like proper walking.)

We have gone beyond this as follows. We found that one doesn't have to use an arm and a leg; just *both sides* of the body — for example, both arms — need be activated. The key is the use of the *precise* arm motion, because if, *AND ONLY IF*, a certain muscle is activated, its corresponding, acupuncture meridian is energized. This in turn is energizing and optimizing to the corresponding *organ*. In this chapter you will learn our Maestro Exercise™ and the Rochlitz Heart Integration Exercise.™ These simple exercises, and indeed, the arm motion performed by music conductors, employ the subscapularis muscle (which lies behind the shoulder blade). This muscle is connected to the heart's acupuncture meridian and in turn to the *heart itself.* So *every time it is used (in the manner we will describe) the heart itself is energized and optimized!*

So we say that this exercise *synchronizes,* or *integrates* the left and right heart hemispheres, and thus strengthens the heart. The use of *both* sides of the body together with the humming (or in some cases counting) gets the brain to re-set, or integrate, or synchronize the heart hemispheres (and the heart's acupuncture meridian.)

This, *at last,* explains the music conductor's arm motion and his/her subsequent journey towards longevity. Music conductor's are coincidentally performing the other aspects our theory states are necessary to insure the success of these special exercises. The music conductor is using both arms, is humming or carrying a tune, and is looking all around at the orchestra! He is performing a Heart Integration™ Exercise! This is a great cardiovascular exercise for all of us. Repeated use apparently continues to keep the heart at an optimum. These exercises may indeed be the best for improving circulation! Athletes report great energy boosts even if they've always had Heart Integration.™ It apparently increases heart output.

CAUTION: If the reader has a disease condition of the heart, kidneys, blood vessels, or related organs, these methods may not work and you should consult your physician first. Get your physician's O.K. if you are not used to doing any exercise. The exercises here need only be performed for a minute or two at first.

Our first *Heart Integration™ Exercise* is called the *MAESTRO EXERCISE.*™ Follow all directions below. See Figure 1.

MAESTRO EXERCISE™[4]

1. Start humming. (A small percentage of people need to do this movement while counting. Do it all the way through *first* while humming. If there is no change, go back and repeat the whole thing while counting out loud.)

2. With the elbows high and out to the side a bit, trace (with your hands) two "C's" that are back to back. The elbows are fairly fixed, only the hands and forearms rotate at the elbow. The hands go down and to the outside; *then bring them back up along the same path.*

3. As you continue this motion, track the perimeter of a large (imaginary) circle with your eyes. The circle is centered around your head. Keep the head facing straight ahead. Rotate only your eyes. If the eye rotation makes you dizzy, *stop it.* Instead, try to substitute the following. Look sequentially at the eight diagonal end- points again centered around your head. See Figure 2.

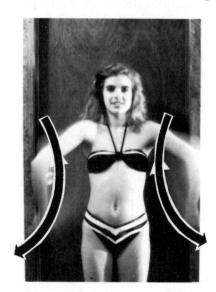

Figure 1.

Maestro Exercise.™ Start with the hands high, elbows up and out and fixed. Bring the hands down & out; then back up and out.

Figure 2.
As you perform the Maestro Exercise,™ look all around the circle *OR*
the *EIGHT outer end-points* of the diagonals.

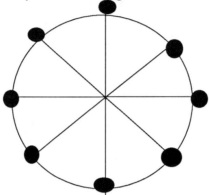

   After a short while, this should flow and not be a jerky one-step-
at-a-time motion. Note that you can do this as slowly as you like,
or while lying down. It will work without rushing it. You should
be relaxed first. If pain or stiffness prevents performance of the
exact recommendations for our Heart Integration Exercises,™ just
do the best you can. It should be fine.

> **STOP READING NOW. PLEASE DO THIS SIMPLE
> CORRECTION NOW. DO IT, IF YOU WANT TO
> INCREASE YOUR LONGEVITY AND YOUR
> HEALTH.**

   Now a music conductor is performing a similar arm movement,
is listening to good music (and may even be counting at the same
time), and is looking all around at the orchestra in front of him/her.
That too is a Heart Integration™ exercise! Once this discovery was
made, it is clear that you don't have to *be* a maestro to *behave* like
one — *or to get the same remarkable benefits.* Indeed, Charlie
Chaplin intrinsically felt this. Often, when listening to classical
music, he would indeed perform the equivalent of our Maestro
Exercise™! He lived to 88. (You can rent the recent video bearing
his name as the title.)
   While performing this special exercise, we track a complete circle,

or the eight diagonal end-points, because this visual activation also activates corresponding parts of the brain (as found by neurobiologists); it helps the whole brain *re-set* this energy circuit. You have a choice of a second Heart Integration Exercise.™ They are roughly equivalent. (The following one may be even better.) We refer to Figures 3 through 6. If you lose your balance here, it is *not* because the exercise is terribly difficult, rather you may have poor balance — a common complaint nowadays. (You can perform any of our remarkable exercises while lying down.) There are other corrections in this book that can help you fix your balance. If, after a minute or two, you are huffing because you don't exercise, maybe it's time to start!

ROCHLITZ HEART INTEGRATION EXERCISE™⁵

1. Start humming. (A small percentage of people may need to perform this exercise while counting. Do it all the way through *first* while humming. If there is no change, go back and repeat the whole thing while counting out loud.)
2. This is a cross-crawl variant; use *opposite* arm and leg. Start out with the right arm as shown in Figure 3.
3. As best as you comfortably can, hold the elbow up at shoulder height and out to the side with the lower arm (and hand) making a right angle with the upper arm. The hand and forearm are pointing down at the floor. This is the scarecrow starting position.
4. Next rotate the arm over to the opposite shoulder. Rotate at the shoulder. (Arm and hand still facing to the floor.).
5. As the elbow reaches the midline, flick up the forearm towards the horizontal or slightly beyond and
6. *Simultaneous with* the right arm flick, bring up the the left knee.
7. Then let them both drop down. That is, the arm drops back to the side while the leg drops to the floor.
8. Repeat with the other pair of opposite arm and leg. Be careful not to do this in a homolateral (same-side) manner.
9. Add the visual, circular tracking (after 30 seconds) as in the first exercise. Use the end points of Figure 2, if you can't track the circle.

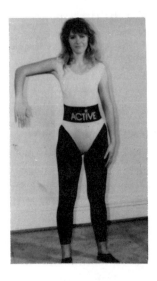
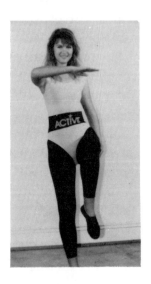
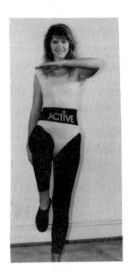
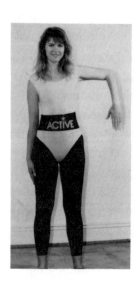

Figures 3 - 6.
Rochlitz Heart Integration™ Exercise. Going clockwise, from the top left: First half starting position, the first half completed, second half starting position, the second half completed.

STOP READING NOW. PLEASE DO THIS SIMPLE CORRECTION NOW. DO IT, IF YOU WANT TO INCREASE YOUR LONGEVITY AND YOUR HEALTH.

After we demonstrate *this* wonderful exercise at lectures or seminars — and get everyone to stand up and do it — we often say, "Now you realize that to get well and live long does *not* have to cost you ... *an arm and a leg!*"

An historical note: The author actually devised this Heart Integration™ Exercise first in 1985 to correct his cardiac arrhythmia. (It did that immediately.) We predicted this would work and would increase our stretch and stamina. It did all that. When a prediction based on an hypothesis works, we have the beginnings of a science! Only a year or so later did we realize that we had uncovered why music conductors have a much greater than expected longevity. Then we revealed the Maestro Exercise.™ We showed that exercise first here because it is easier to do for most people, even though this one may be even more powerful.

But, back in 1985, this author discovered that *the heart hemispheres can become "dyslexic."* We coined the term *"dyslexic heart"*[6] because the heart hemispheres are not functioning *together* properly if this condition occurs. This is analogous to dyslexia where the two brain hemispheres are not working together properly. (See chapter eight.) With dyslexic heart, the heart is out of "synche" with itself and the brain. This condition may not show up on an EKG (Electrocardiogram), as dyslexia does not show up on EEG tests. (Recent computerized, statistical interpretations of EEG's do *at last* reveal a dyslexic profile.[7] Perhaps one day this author's discovery of dyslexic heart will also be observed similarly on an advanced EKG.) We sometimes say that our simple Exercises *correct*, or *prevent*, "dyslexic heart." This is why we call them "Heart Integration™ Exercises."

A final word on humming versus counting. The majority of the time, it is sufficient to do these special exercises while *humming*. (This helps activate the *right* brain hemisphere.) Take deep breaths and deeply hum out as you do our "arm jogging." Sometimes the problem is in the left hemisphere, so counting is needed. You can even cover all bases, by singing a song of numbers to duplicate how a conductor may numerically keep tempo while conducting the music.

In addition to leading to a greater life-span as many music conductors enjoy, you may find the following complaints are improved: Cold hands and feet, bruising, pale complexion, faulty blood pressure (low or high), cardiac arrhythmias, "frozen joints," varicose veins, muscular or joint stiffness and achiness. If you have cardiac arrhythmia for no medical reason, you may likely benefit, but you should know that (hidden) allergies are often the cause of this complaint. In fact, Arthur Coca, M.D., created the Coca pulse test which demonstrates that the heart rate changes (often speeding up) from allergic reactions. (Take your pulse before and after eating suspected food allergies. Don't eat anything that you know will make you very ill! Take your pulse every five minutes afterwards and write this all down. Within an hour or so you should note the change.) Many people know that they have missing heartbeats or "ectopics."

Some holistic physicians routinely treat cold hands and feet with thyroid medication. (Sometimes, appropriate testing isn't done.) This may not always be relevant as we now know!

After performing either of these two Heart Integration Exercises, ™ you may feel stronger, more energetic and even less foggy. But this will be a subtle feeling; *not* like getting a shot of caffeine. This exercise is perhaps the most important correction for those with M.S. (Mulitple Sclerosis), or *anyone* that has problems on *one side* of the body worse than the other.

It helps to have "hard evidence" and we do have it. First we've seen it normalize, or at least lower, high blood pressure in *minutes*. This is remarkable since any exercise tends to raise blood pressure. We have the printouts as proof. (See the last page of Chapter 7 — on blood pressure.) It will also usually normalize (raise) low blood pressure.

Figure 7.

The leg
abduction
test.

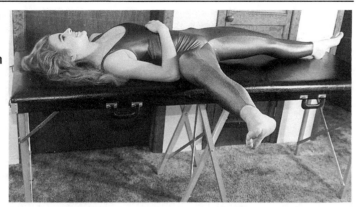

Another visual "proof" is the following. Here, we make use of changes in leg abduction (spreading apart). With your subject lying on a table or the floor, mark (below, on the floor) the exact spot that they can abduct (spread) a leg out to the side, stopping at the point when pain begins. Constrain the non-moving leg. (See Figure 7.) Mark the big toe's position (vertically down to the floor.) Also note where the head and hips were. You want to make sure you put the subject back in the same starting position. If the person is on a table, mark the spot vertically below their big toe. Use the leg that has *more circulatory difficulty* for this procedure. After either Heart Integration™ Exercise is performed, retest the leg abduction. See where the leg moves out to now. Mark this on the floor as before. We've seen changes of six inches to three feet! (Changes of less than three inches are insignificant.)

Even those with "great stretches" show marked improvement. One dancer was finally able to wrap her leg around her neck. See Figure 8 which is a picture of a student in our Advanced Seminar in 1987. The class thought that Rochlitz found the wrong subject to demonstrate the effects of Heart Integration™ on. This person could already stretch either leg out to the side so far that it lined up vertically! She is a dancer and international dance choreographer. She informed us that one stretch she could never do was to put her foot over and behind her neck. After performing the exercise, this author said, "well, you're heart's integrated now, so try it now."

Figure 8.

A demonstration
of increased
stretch.

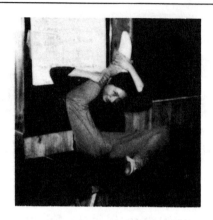

We immediately snapped a Polaroid of the result![8]

How could this happen? Answer: If the adductor muscle in the leg stretches much better, it can only mean that it has a better supply of blood. But — since we did nothing special to *this* one muscle — this must be true of the entire body! Many feel their hands warming up within seconds or minutes. Others feel more comfortable, or less achy, in their seats, suddenly.

This is not necessarily a permanent correction. *If* dietary factors — described in Chapter 7 — are involved, and the offending foods are not eliminated, this correction may not last long. Do it everyday for as long as you can, just like music conductors (who conduct for up to hours at a time.) As it is virtually devoid of side-effects, we recommend you do it for, at least, two minutes a day for the rest of your long life!

A variation of this exercise may have been known in the former Soviet Union. Most troops march in cross-crawl fashion, with the swinging arm either coming straight up or going towards the opposite knee. On old, Soviet films of their May Day, (or new ones of the Russian May Day), you can see these troops march with the arm making a similar flick up to the opposite side as we do in the Rochlitz Heart Integration™ Exercise. (Of course the gun prevents utilizing the opposite pair of limbs. And they don't start out with the optimum scarecrow position.)

The elderly often need to do these Heart Integration Exercises™

to regain their health. We hope cardiologists and gerontologists will contact us about the use of our discoveries for their patients. These Heart Integration™ Exercises are great to do before any strenuous activity and some people may have intrinsically felt this. You can rent the video of the movie, *THE MUSIC MAN*; watch Robert Preston march while flicking his opposite arm much like the Rochlitz Heart Integration™ Exercise!

Let's end our discussion of Heart Integration™ with another discovery. We have realized that the connection of the heart to the muscle used in our corrective exercises is intuitively realized by many societies and seems to be *inherent in children*. We've seen African tribal greeting and parting ceremonies. These dances contain arm waving that clearly uses the heart muscles. And how does a baby wave good-bye? Yes, it's from the heart! See Figure 9.

Figure 9.

Saying good-bye from
the heart.

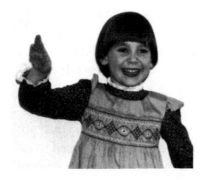

3

BREAKTHROUGH FOR LIVING TO YOUR 120'S? — BEYOND THE MAESTRO!

If the Rochlitz Heart Integration Exercises™ *duplicate* the major factor responsible for music conductors' longevities, is it possible to go *beyond* this? Can our understanding of this phenomenon suggest further improvements that can lead to even greater longevity and benefits in cardiovascular function?

We believe the answer is a resounding *"yes."* The author's breakthrough understanding of neurological disorganization, Applied Kinesiology and acupuncture theory led, in 1987, to his formulation of Meta-Integration™ Exercises.[9] These exercises utilize a simultaneous, *four-limbed* motion. They are harder to do, more easily interfered with (or switched off), and even *more beneficial* (once they are "switched on") than are the two-limbed Heart Integration™ exercises we devised.

CAUTION: If the reader has a disease condition of the heart, kidneys, blood vessels, or related organs, these methods may not work and you should consult your physician first. Get your physician's O.K., if you are not used to doing any exercising.

Obviously we can't yet prove gains in longevity because this unique motion has only been performed by our students for six years or so. But there are ways to demonstrate that this exercise produces results even greater than those from the two-limbed Heart Integration Exercises.™ One such method is to use the leg abduction shown in the last chapter (Figure 7). Having marked off where the increased stretch from the two-limbed Heart Integration Exercises™ was made; you will undoubtedly see an even greater increase in stretch after performing the Meta-Maestro™ Exercise shown below. Indeed, for all the purposes outlined in this book, we assert the Meta-Maestro™ Exercise will provide greater benefit than the two-limbed corrections. For increasing longevity, normalizing blood pressure, increasing stretch and stamina, overcoming fatigue and for many other purposes, the Meta-Maestro™ Exercise will provide greater improvement, and just as rapidly as did the two-limbed corrections. You can — once you have mastered them all — perform only this last, best one if you like. Or you can alternate them as your mood suggests.

You might want to re-familiarize yourself with the Maestro Exercise™ from the last chapter. This next one, we called the Meta-Maestro™ because "Meta" means "beyond" and we are going beyond the music conductors' centuries-old, two-armed correction which has helped them attain great longevity! As before, this exercise can be done lying down if there is a problem doing it standing up. You can do this as slowly as you like. It will work without rushing it. You should be relaxed first.

META-MAESTRO™ EXERCISE[10]

1. Start, and continue, humming throughout. (In some cases, people need to count. First do it completely through with the hum. If you feel or see no improvement, go back and try this while counting out loud.)
2. With the elbows high and out to the side a bit, trace (with your hands, not your eyes) two "C's" that are back to back.
3. Add the circular, visual tracking or look at the diagonal end points (as before). So far this is just the Maestro Exercise.™
4. Now move your legs in and out to the rhythm of your hands. This is a variation of "jumping jacks." Start with your hands high and feet together. See Figure 10. As the hands come down and to the outside your feet will jump to the outside. See Figure 11.
5. As the hands go back up and towards themselves and then to the outside, the feet will jump back together again. Back to Figure 10.

6. Keep repeating steps 1-5 for two minutes in a continuous fashion. After a short while, this should flow and not be a jerky one step-at-a-time motion.

**Figures 10 &
11.**
Meta-Maestro
Exercise.™

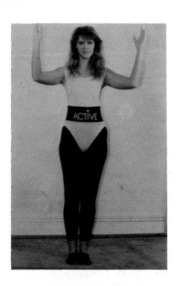 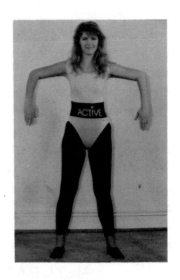

STOP READING NOW! PLEASE DO THIS SIMPLE CORRECTION NOW! DO IT, IF YOU WANT TO INCREASE YOUR LONGEVITY AND YOUR HEALTH.

This is the most powerful of all three Rochlitz Heart Integration™ Exercises. Indeed, it's on another level. This is because the use of all four limbs attains or corrects neurological disorganization on a higher plane. Maybe it can help you make it to your 120's! That's if you follow the diet, nutrition and other recommendations in this book.

4

THE DIET CONNECTION
FOR LIVING TO YOUR 90'S

If we want to make it into our 90's and beyond, we will have to make certain diet changes. You will see that with our diet breakthroughs, it's also possible to be physically and mentally healthy into your 90's and beyond. Dispelling various common, diet myths is also one of this chapter's goals, as is realizing that accepted medical dogma often emphasizes the wrong things.

There are certain foods that you should avoid, or minimize, if longevity is your goal. Just performing our Heart Integration Exercises™ while we eat the wrong foods may not maximize our longevities. Indeed, the improvements made by these novel Heart Integration Exercises™ may not last if we poison our bodies with the wrong foods!

We'll start with the obvious. Avoid all tobacco products. Some allergists demonstrated decades ago, that tobacco causes a spasm of the arteries[11] that feed the heart itself. They understood this to be a type of allergic reaction. This is in addition to the toxic effects of nicotine and carbon monoxide that are in smoked tobacco. Due to the nicotine and the allergic response just noted, chewing tobacco will not eliminate the threat to your life. Avoid all tobacco, period.

The next great, and commonly used, stressor to the heart and circulatory system is caffeine. This is one of the western world's great (and still unrecognized) addictions. Caffeine can be found in coffee, tea, cola and chocolate. Caffeine constricts the blood vessels and stresses the adrenal glands, pancreas and liver. We have also found caffeine to be more addictive than nicotine for many people! Indeed, Coca Cola® got its name a century ago because it contained small amounts of another great, addictive, cardiac stressor — cocaine. But caffeine is probably more addictive! Our society bears this out. How many people do you know that can get by without coffee, tea or cola on a daily basis? Many people cannot quit nicotine unless they *first* quit caffeine. As is the nature of the *allergy/addiction syndrome,* the person that says s/he can't get started in the morning without his/her caffeine is describing a person who is addicted and needs the *next fix* to overcome the withdrawal — *the result of the last fix!* All such people, if they ever go a week without their caffeine, will report a much higher and *steadier* level of energy throughout their day. This will be without the up and down, energy-level (and mood) swings. It will be without the mid-afternoon sleepiness from caffeine-induced low blood sugar (hypoglycemia). There will be far less of the anxieties, phobias and nervousness that caffeineholics experience. A large percentage of western society is addicted to caffeine. Sadly, we've seen babies, even infants, left to wean themselves on bottles of cola. A lifetime of addiction and misery thus begins.

We're sure you probably haven't heard of at least one property of caffeinated substances. Through the author's knowledge of Applied Kinesiology and acupuncture meridians, we have discovered that caffeine can freeze the acupuncture meridians that energize the heart and/or the adrenal glands. When you are young, this will have the effect of constantly over-energizing you. You may feel nervous much of the time. As the susceptible person ages, these meridians and organs can get frozen in an *under-energized state.* You will then suffer from frequent or chronic fatigue. An expert kinesiologist may be needed to unfreeze these meridians. Or, our special exercises may do just that. If your caffeine withdrawal is very bad, it implies that caffeine was a severe allergen or toxin to your body.

"Decaffeinated coffee" or tea is still dangerous on at least two accounts. First there will be several per cent caffeine remaining; and caffeine, as we said, is also a very, common allergy (even in small amounts.) Secondly, unless water (steam) is used to do the de-caffeinating, a toxic, carcinogenic substance is often used instead. For the sake of your longevity, learn to drink pure water primarily. Many people will deride this suggestion because their tap water tastes so bad (from chlorine, fluoride, etc) that they think water was meant to taste like that. Try some bottled, spring water first. If you live in the country, you may even have a nearby spring where you can bottle-up for free. Try to buy spring water in the newer, thicker, clear plastic (or glass) bottles. Then, after you taste the difference, buy a good water purifier. Some fine choices include devices with a reverse osmosis element or a heavy carbon block. Make all your beverages, herb teas and soups from pure water. Everything will taste better and you'll be healthier. You can substitute herb teas for the caffeinated kind. Health stores, and now even supermarkets, carry many different varieties of herb teas. Sample them all. Look for the words "No caffeine" and *not* "de-caffeinated." And don't drink all your pure water in carbonated form as some people do. Too much carbonation can make your body too acidic and the excess pressure in the stomach can cause problems in some people.

The next class of foods to avoid for the sake of your health and longevity is dairy. Dairy products, including milk, cheese, yoghurt, and butter, have long been infamous (in knowledgeable circles) for causing gastrointestinal and circulatory ills. More recently, studies have shown they can be toxic to the pancreas and lead to diabetes.[12] In this last instance, you may recall the recent press conference called by celebrated "baby doctor," Benjamin Spock, M.D.[13]

Simply put, pasteurized, homogenized, cow's milk products are among the worst foods one could eat. Don't be fooled by the earlier nutritionists' dogma that milk is a "natural" substance and must be good. It is *unnatural* for man to consume these milk products! In nature, a mammal ingests *only* its mother's milk and *only* in its infancy. Whether or not it comes from a machine is not a viable definition of unnatural! The proteins (casein, lactalbumin, whey) found even in raw milk can be toxic and allergenic. The molds found in milk and cheese are capable of causing health problems.

These molds are a leading cause of high blood pressure as we shall see in the chapter on high blood pressure. Most adults will eventually develop intolerance to the sugars — lactose and galactose — found in milk. Lactose intolerance can be due to milk allergy. The homogenization and pasteurization process is also said to create the enzyme, xanthine oxidase. In large amounts, this substance is toxic to the blood vessels and initiates cardiovascular illness. Autopsies of 18 year-old Americans killed in Vietnam revealed the blood vessels of eighty year-olds. Xanthine oxidase from dairy products is the suspected cause. In Europe, raw goat's milk products are used with better results. This still contains lactose, molds, and similar proteins to cow's milk though. Commercial dairy products may even be a poor source of calcium. Raw milk contains an enzyme which splits calcium from the phosphorus it's bound to. Pasteurization destroys this enzyme; so humans may not be able to utilize the calcium in milk. Do not trust any nutritional "news" that may have been sponsored by a grant from the dairy industry! Also fat-free milk is usually no less harmful as it still contains toxic or allergenic proteins and undigestible sugars. It's not the fat that is the worst culprit in milk.

It's never too early to start the quest for longevity. Help your children (or grandchildren) by seeing to it that mother's milk is what they get! It is certainly best for infants. (There is one proviso. The baby may suffer if the mother doesn't avoid foods that *she* is allergic to! Undigested, allergenic proteins can enter her milk and affect the infant.)

Milk is alkaline or basic — the opposite of acidic. Alkalinity counteracts acidity — such as in an ulcerous stomach. This was the rationale for gastroenterologists to put their ulcer patients on a milk diet. Most now know better. Gastric (stomach), allergic reactions lead to histamine, and subsequent acid, release. But milk, being alkaline, can counteract its own acid release — *temporarily.* Hours later though, an acid or sour stomach can still result. We often say, "Show me someone who wakes up with a sour stomach, and I'll show you someone who got high drinking milk the night before."

Now if a food (like milk) causes gastrointestinal and pancreatic irritation or inflammation, its nutrients will not be well absorbed. The irritation can lower absorbability of nutrients from other foods for *days*. Therefore, *the allergenicity of a food takes precedence over its theoretical, nutritive value.* Chronic gastrointestinal irritation from eating allergic foods or from eating too much food is a leading cause of malnutrition in affluent or civilized(?) societies.

Sugar (sucrose) is another food to avoid. Contrary to medical dogma, evidence exists that dietary sugar and dairy products, and *not dietary* cholesterol, are the cause of the cholesterol buildup in the arteries. To understand this, we first need to learn something about cholesterol. Despite its bad reputation, its purpose is to coat the blood vessels, thus facilitating the flow of blood in the blood vessels. The body produces more cholesterol than almost anybody can eat! So clearly it is not the cholesterol in food (dietary cholesterol) that is the culprit in the improper metabolism of cholesterol that leads to its build-up against the blood vessel walls. We will further prove this assertion in the next chapter when we refer to the high cholesterol (blubber) diet of Eskimos who have a remarkably low incidence of cardiovascular disease.

Dairy products and *sugar* are the two leading dietary factors that actually can cause the body to improperly metabolize cholesterol which starts its build-up in the arteries. If you must use a sweetener, try maple syrup, rice syrup or honey. Skip the cakes, sodas, cookies, and ice cream that have an abundance of sugar in them. Recognize if you're a sugarholic. Learn to be honest with yourself about your addictions. This is the first step in eliminating them. The sugarholic will say, "I can't eat the heath food store ice cream that is sweetened with rice syrup, honey or fruit juice. *It has to be sugar.*" Here is the allergy/addiction syndrome again. Your favorite foods are the ones to which you are really allergic and addicted to.

Some foods contain a class of chemicals called monoamines.[14] They are vasoactive — they affect the diameter of blood vessels. (We believe any allergic food can do this.) Monoamines are found in cheese, wine, anything fermented, coffee, chocolate, citrus, beans, bananas. Avoiding foods with monoamines can lead to a normalization of high blood pressure within days of changing the diet! (There will be a further discussion of monoamines in chapter 7.)

Getting back to cholesterol, if you do not follow the diet and supplement recommendations made in this book, eating foods with high cholesterol may indeed worsen the cholesterol build-up in your arteries. Red meats are worst here. But meats are also very bad on other accounts. Most standard American meats are laden with artificial (and potentially carcinogenic) hormones, antibiotics, tranquilizers and other toxic chemicals. New Zealand and Argentine meats are best. They are often organic. At the end of the Reagan administration in the U.S., several European countries banned the importation of American meats, not as a nationalistic practice, but because of the toxins they contain. (This didn't stop Reagan from retaliating in a nationalistic way by banning certain European cheeses and wines. Maybe everyone benefitted!)

Avoid alcoholic beverages to increase your longevity and to have a healthy circulatory system. Ignore "research" that claims wine everyday is good for you. (Read the small print and find that the wine industry financed these studies.) Alcoholic beverages are laden with mold, monoamines, sulfites, acetaldehyde (similar but more toxic than formaldehyde) and other toxins to your circulatory system.

Try to avoid microwaved foods, nuts and seeds that may be rancid, and foods cooked in heated oils. All these substances contain *free radicals* or oxidized substances. (Bake or broil with a minimum, or absence, of oil.) Free radicals are *highly reactive* substances. They have an unpaired electron, and, by the laws of physics, are desperate to find another electron by attaching to anything. The free radical can damage any molecule or cell that it attaches to. Free radical damage has been known for some time to be part of aging theory. The dangerous, lipid peroxide radicals are found in all heated or rancid oils and in other substances. Many nuts and seeds, by the time you can buy them, have gone partially rancid and thus are full of free radicals. (The chapter on supplements contains a list of nutrients — anti-oxidants — that help combat free radicals.) But, nothing works as well as prevention; try not to eat these foods. If you want the speed of a microwave oven, without its dangerous free radicals, buy a convection oven or the new portable, electric, glass cookers that move air over all the food at high speed. They cook as fast as microwaves without creating free radicals. Our research indicates that food cooked in these devices tastes great too.

Likewise, avoid margarine as its *hydrogenated oils* are similar, in their dangerous and aging properties, to the heated oils noted above. Here is another example of something (butter) getting a bad reputation (somewhat deservedly), yet replaced by something worse.

Avoid eating chicken unless it's absolutely, organically raised — without the use of hormones, antibiotics and other chemicals. We know you've been told to avoid red meats and may be eating a lot of chicken at this time. But the pioneering cancer researcher, Virginia Livingston Wheeler, M.D. demonstrated that chicken contains the *Progenitor cryptocides* germ. She proved that this germ causes cancer.[15] (She deserves a Nobel Prize for her work.) Turkey apparently does not contain this dangerous germ.

Avoiding cancer is one of the goals of this book and of anyone who wants a long and healthy life. Avoiding chicken and foods with free radicals, eating a high fiber diet, and taking the anti-oxidant nutrients listed in the next chapter will go a long way towards preventing cancer — the second leading cause of death in the Western world.

Start buying organic produce. Pesticides are far more dangerous than the chemical industry wants you to know. Most are neurotoxic to insects. (It destroys their nerve cells.) But a human nerve cell is very similar to an insect's. Research has appeared in the scientific journals for nearly a decade now indicating that pesticides may be the cause of most degenerative, neurological disease. This includes Parkinson's and Alzheimer's Diseases.[16] The purpose of this book is not just to enable you to increase your chances for longevity, but to provide you with great mental and physical health and well-being all the days of your life. Health food stores, some local produce stands in the country, and even some supermarkets sell organically grown fruits and vegetables. They taste better too!

Processed foods contain much pesticide as wells as artificial colors, flavors, preservatives and sweeteners. Many of these artificial ingredients are allowed in only one country — the USA. France has allowed only about a dozen of these substances in their foods while the U.S. allows over 5,000. Just as we're sure that one day all artificial pesticides will be banned, so too will many of these artificial ingredients.

The artificial sweetener, aspartame, will likely be eventually banned too. It has a drastic effect on memory and other neurological functions.[17] Avoid it, if you want to have a working memory into your 90's!

MSG (monosodium glutamate) adversely affects many susceptible people. Headaches, asthma, and cardiovascular crises are among its many possible symptoms. When eating out, always insist your chef avoid all MSG. We have found that many cooks making all kinds of cuisines — not just Chinese food — use MSG. Beware! Of course, when you eat out, the cook may likely use heated oils (frying or grilling) or a microwave. Foods seared on a grill or barbecue have also been found to contain some carcinogens. (A high intake of Vitamins C and A may help counteract these, however.)

If you or your family elders are arthritic, try to avoid nightshades which include tomatoes (and tomato sauce), potatoes, eggplants, peppers and tobacco. Tomatoes are the worst here. The ancient, Greek, medical literature said that tomatoes were a poison and the western world followed this decree for nearly two millennia. Now there is much arthritis in our senior citizens! Other foods — if you are allergic to them — can also cause arthritis. Some additional likely culprits are citrus fruits, dairy products and wheat. Get individual allergy testing if you have arthritis or try elimination diets and make a food diary. List foods, symptoms and times; you'll likely find your culprits.

No one, of course, can follow all these recommendations perfectly. Just use them as guidelines and do the best you can. Ignorance is not bliss as far as your health and longevity are concerned. Do eat lots of fresh, (preferably) organic vegetables and fruits. (If you have blood sugar problems, many allergies, or a Candida-Yeast problem [see Appendix A], you may have to go easy on the fruits.) If you eat fish, try to purchase those that comes from unpolluted waters. Shellfish live at the coastline where much pollution is dumped, and should be eaten minimally at best. Fresh water fish from unpolluted lakes may be fine for you. Avoid fish from waters that have been found high in PCB's, or mercury or other toxic, heavy metals. Pay attention to your local and national news sources for this information as it changes.

Do eat foods high in fiber at every meal. Rice and millet are usually the best tolerated grains. Wheat and corn are usually the least tolerated. Oats, rye and barley lie in between. Eat anything else such as beans and root vegetables that you tolerate. Avoid eating the same foods every day. These are likely your allergy/addiction foods! Take a long, slow walk all around your supermarket or health food store. Observe and purchase some *new* foods and enjoy.

EATING TIPS

Yes, eating can, and should, still be fun! The following tips begin with our repeating some of the "obvious." Avoid allergic foods. Avoid eating safe foods too frequently as they *may become* allergenic. Don't eat when under physical or emotional stress. Eat in ecologically sound environments. Have good air, lighting, (classical) music, friends and other ambient conditions. You can eat shortly after exercising as this often prevents reactions unless you are in the stressful, building-up phase of exercising. Don't overeat as many Americans do. Four to six ounces of protein daily should be sufficient for most adults. Overeating can stress your detoxifying organs (such as your kidneys) and actually lead to malnourishment. Try a vegetarian diet to see if it works for you. Many people do well on it, but due to allergies and genetic intolerances (such as

some people have with beans), it may not be for everyone. Do cut
down on meats, as many meat-eaters ingest too high a percentage
of calories from protein and fat. Your kidneys, gall bladder and
other organs could be stressed if you overeat meats. Try to get most
of your calories from complex carbohydrates (starchy foods) that
you can safely eat.

If you are hypoglycemic (which may self-correct if you do everything in this book), eat frequent, small meals. This is also less
stressful to the digestive system. Don't drink while eating as this
dilutes the digestive enzymes. Do drink plenty of good water 45
minutes before, and an hour after, eating. Drink eight glasses of
pure water a day. Always be on guard for new cravings. Chew your
food very well. Avoid raw or undercooked meats and fish. Bacteria
and parasites are the danger here. Avoid chopped meats as these
have a high surface area of exposure for bacteria and molds. Avoid
excess sodium. Though not an allergy as such, it can lead to edema,
dehydration, and has even been linked to cancer. (Craving salt may
be a sign of adrenal exhaustion.) Cook and serve food *only* in glass,
porcelain, cast iron and stainless steel. Do learn, and abide by,
FOOD COMBINING guidelines. See Figure 12.

As we age, our digestive organs will decline in function. Food
combining will become increasingly important. Basically, fruits
should be eaten alone. Likewise for heavy protein or fatty foods.
You may be able to get away with some complex carbohydrate at

Non-starchy & green vegetables—goes with any food includes: green leafy veggies, cabbage, lettuce, celery, etc.
Starchy vegetables—with green salad, not with protein or fruit includes: potato, corn, squash, coconut, artichoke, carrot
Proteins—with salads, not with starch or fruits includes: meats, sprouts, beans, nuts, seeds, grains
Melons—alone, or avoid if have Candida
Sub-acid fruits —only with either acid or sweet fruits includes: papaya, mango, apple, pear, cherry, berries, grapes, peach
Acid fruits—only with sub-acid fruits

Figure 12. Food Combining Guidelines.

the same meal. Test this experientially as some cannot. You can eat green vegetables with almost anything. If you will not be at home, have safe foods prepared *ahead of time*. Avoid cheating binges. Don't hate yourself if one starts, just get back on track.

Obviously no one can stick to all these diet guidelines 100% of the time. Do the best you can.

SUMMARY OF FOODS, ETC.
TO AVOID FOR YOUR LONGEVITY
Tobacco
Caffeine
Dairy Products
Sugar
Foods Containing monoamines
Excess meats
Ground or Undercooked meats
Alcoholic Beverages
Microwaved Foods
Foods Cooked In Heated Oils
Rancid Nuts & Seeds
Non-organic Chicken
Margarine
Foods With pesticides
Foods With Artificial Color, Flavor, Preservatives
MSG (Monosodium Glutamate)
Nightshades (tomatoes, potatoes, eggplants, peppers) if arthritic
Aspartame (the artificial sweetener)

GOOD FOODS SUMMARY
Vegetables
Some Fruits (Based On Individuality)
Some Grains (Rice, Millet Are Often Best, Oats May Be Good)
High Fiber
Fish
Turkey
Many Foods Not Prohibited In the List Above

5

NUTRITIONAL SUPPLEMENTS FOR LIVING TO YOUR 90'S

If we want to live into our 90's and beyond, we may have to take various nutrients to help us attain this goal. The circulatory system needs large amounts of nutrients to function properly. Contrary to standard, medical dogma, you will probably *not* get enough of many of these nutrients in your diet! Let's examine some of the many reasons why supplementation is often needed for optimum wellness and for increasing our longevities.

A nutritional deficiency may be at the root of a medical condition or a "sub-clinical" complaint. Thus wellness cannot be attained *without* supplementation. Emotional and physical stress have also been proven to deplete nutrients. Most foods eaten are deficient in many nutrients for the following reasons: Abuse and overuse of the soil, use of fertilizers, pesticides, freezing, canning and processing of food, loss during transportation, and loss during cooking. How many eat only organic foods just plucked from the ground as nature intended? Certain crucial microminerals, like the cancer-fighting selenium, are almost completely depleted from much soil. Some say supplementation leads to expensive urine and is thus a waste. But who would say paying insurance premiums for your house is a waste just because it hasn't *yet* burned down! And expensive urine is a lot cheaper than paying for the expensive physicians that say such things to their patients *after* they've gotten sick. Yes, the facts support the need for supplementation.

It is especially appropriate to discuss some nutrients in this book. These special micro-nutrients can greatly improve our cardiovascular functioning.

CARDIOVASCULAR NUTRIENTS

VITAMINS:
VITAMIN E
VITAMIN C
VITAMIN P (Bioflavonoids)
VITAMIN B3
VITAMIN B6
FISH OIL-MAX-EPA® (VITAMIN F)
MINERALS:
MAGNESIUM
POTASSIUM
SELENIUM
SILICON
AMINO ACIDS:
CARNITINE
TAURINE
OTHER NUTRIENTS
LECITHIN
COENZYME Q10
MUCOPOLYSACCHARIDES

Let's see why our hearts have to have these nutrients if we are to make it to our 90's and beyond. In 1993, the major media finally revealed the amazing properties of Vitamin E. Drs. Wilfred and Evan Shute, of Canada, however, proved these matters three decades ago when the pharmaceutical/medical establishment still refused to even acknowledge that Vitamin E was a Vitamin. Vitamin E helps prevent cardiovascular disease, including heart attacks, and it is a powerful anti-oxidant especially against fatty free radicals (such as lipid peroxides). This vitamin can help clear carbon monoxide from the blood. It works well with selenium and is recommended to be taken without iron. Vitamin E occurs in *fresh, whole* grains and vegetable oils, nuts, seeds and soybeans. Earlier, we noted that foods high in oil are often rancid by the time they're sold and eaten. The Vitamin E in these foods — which can prevent rancidity — will *itself* go rancid if these foods are not fresh, whole and raw. So supplementation from a reputable manufacturer of supplements can be crucial here. (Avoid companies that describe themselves only as "distributors," instead of *"manufacturers"* on their labels. By the time, you'd be ingesting it, years could have passed since this vitamin was manufactured.)

The Recommended Daily Allowance (RDA) of Vitamin E is about 15 IU (International Units) for adults. Most medical nutritionists recommend at least 100 IU daily, with a gradual build-up to 400 IU daily. Its sources in supplements include wheat (if the Vitamin E is listed as natural and not declared to have any other source), soy, and synthetic derivatives.

Vitamin C can remove plaque build-up from the walls of our arteries. It also is crucial for capillary strength and the formation of red blood cells. We will have more to say about Vitamin C in the anti-oxidant section later in this chapter. Vitamin P, the bioflavonoids, works with Vitamin C for capillary strength too. We'll also have more on this nutrient later in this chapter.

The niacin form of Vitamin B3 has powerful, anti-cholesterol effects and is even used by mainstream physicians. It can cause a "flush." If you take a large amount, say over a 100 mg. (milligrams), you may get the flush. In a flush, joints and other areas of your body will turn red, and get hot, as your blood vessels dilate (widen) from the niacin. Drinking a lot of water can help end this effect. Or you can take smaller amounts. Time-release forms are also recommended by physicians and nutritionists.

Vitamin B6 (pyridoxine) is needed for formation of blood cells, hormones, neurotransmitters, enzymes, and antibodies. It can reduce edema. We'll have more to say about this Vitamin later in the chapter.

Eskimos have very little cardiovascular disease despite their high fish blubber diet. The blubber has a *very, high cholesterol content.* But it also contains EPA (Eicosapentanoic acid). This nutrient, a form of Vitamin F, or essential fatty acid, thus is known to prevent cardiovascular disease. Mackerel and salmon are high in this form of Vitamin F. The supplement is called Max-EPA®.

Now for your heart's necessary minerals. Magnesium is crucial here. Clots in the heart and brain can result from inadequate magnesium intake.[18] It is also used to counter cardiac arrhythmias. Excess calcium induces a magnesium deficiency. Take as much magnesium as calcium.

Potassium is crucial for regulation of the heartbeat. Diuretic drugs often cause a depletion of this crucial nutrient, and other necessary minerals. Excess sodium induces a potassium deficiency. Avoid eating processed, salty food. You can buy a salt substitute that is potassium chloride instead of sodium chloride. Don't overdo this either, as a great amount of potassium can slow down the heartbeat.

Selenium helps insure that the heart muscle itself will receive an adequate oxygen supply by optimizing the heart's energy-producing cells. It also helps prevent platelet aggregation in the blood vessels. Silicon is needed for all structural tissues including the heart itself.

The amino acid, carnitine helps transport fatty acids across our cells' energy factories — the mitochondria. After a heart attack, carnitine levels, in the heart, often drop to *zero,* making it crucial for the sufferer!

Deficiency of taurine (an amino acid) can cause cardiac arrhythmia, epilepsy, insomnia and excessive jerking while in the act of falling asleep. Taurine is also needed to make bile. The kidneys may spill taurine if you eat too much meat.

Lecithin is a great emulsifier of fats and cholesterol. Eggs are very high in lecithin, and therefore are *not* bad for you, unless you are allergic to them, contrary to medical dogma. Soybean is also high in lecithin. Lecithin contains choline which is needed to form the neurotransmitter, acetylcholine. Deficiencies, or disorders, of this transmitter have been linked to degenerative, neurological diseases. Research on Coenzyme Q_{10} has shown that it significantly increases oxygen uptake in heart cells. The heart can then tolerate more stress of any kind. It is so beneficial for the cardiovascular system that the U.S. FDA (Food and Drug Administration) wants to ban it! Apparently, if a *safe* nutrient — naturally occurring in the body — can replace an expensive and *patented* (read immensely profitable) drug, the FDA will come down on it! Coenzyme Q_{10} is available as a supplement beginning in 10 mg. amounts.

Mucopolysaccharides are a class of nutrients that are also beneficial for the cardiovascular system. They include carageenan (from seaweed) or chondroitin sulfate A (CSA) from beef aorta tissue. These are available as supplements.

Now we need to understand the effects of aging (or of eating the wrong foods) on our digestive abilities. The elderly are often put on antacids when in fact they need to *augment* low stomach acidity by taking supplements with pepsin and betaine hydrochloride. Low stomach acidity allows things to ferment and this then causes pain; *thus the stomach ache.* Here, mainstream medicine is doing precisely the *opposite* of what they should be doing to help people. We have found that this very common condition of low stomach acidity is often initiated by eating dairy, caffeine or sugar. In addition to pain, this condition may cut down on the ability to absorb nutrients.

You can indirectly test your stomach's ability to produce sufficient acid. You can buy pH paper from your laboratory supply company (in the yellow pages) or drug store. Saliva pH supposedly mirrors intestinal pH and should be around 7.5. Urine pH mirrors the stomach's pH, and it (the urine) should be around 5.5. If it's much higher, say 7.0, it usually means your stomach is not producing enough acid, and you should consider a pepsin/hydrochloride supplement. (People with ulcers should never take acid supplements.) Correct low stomach acidity as needed with your nutritionist's advice.

Be wary of books that recommend many hundreds of milligrams of B-vitamins. Note that, some nutrients, e.g. iron and copper oxidize (literally, rust) readily. These, unless you are anemic or pregnant, are usually not needed in supplements. The body also stores these two nutrients fairly well. Many nutrients *may* be needed, at some time, in smaller amounts, as blood and other tests indicate. You can never be tested too much!

Though we recommend nutritional support, this should never be done unconditionally. Though far less dangerous than drugs, there are points to be made aware of. Many allow supplements to spoil by letting them sit too long or allowing them to heat up or get too cold. If you are allergic to a supplement, get rid of it. Many companies use overkill. While their capsules may have one or two safe nutrients, the company feels they have to be "one up" on their competition; so they add an additional dozen ingredients. Less can definitely be more here. Add enough ingredients and people will likely be allergic to one or more of them. Get only what you need. But, there are hardly any life-threatening dangers to supplementing, unlike pharmaceutical prescribing. Hypoallergenic supplements are obtainable.

A NOTE ON ASPIRIN

There is much more to the study that is the basis of the daily aspirin recommendation than the medical establishment would like you to know.[19] First off, the participants in the one study on American male, medical physicians — while allegedly having a lesser incidence of heart attacks — had an *increased* incidence of *strokes*. Also, a similar, British study found *no decrease* in heart attacks from daily aspirin ingestion; but the increased incidence of strokes *did* show up! And the alleged decrease in heart attacks, from the first study, may not have been due to aspirin. This is because the usual acetylsalicylic acid form of aspirin was not used. Instead the *magnesium salicylate* form was used. The additional magnesium may have been the factor that led to the supposed decrease in heart attacks as magnesium is known to have this property.

The medical recommendation of daily ingestion of aspirin to prevent heart attacks is part of a larger enterprise. The collusion between the medical and pharmaceutical industries has led to the

warped dogmas of "vitamins as drugs" and "drugs as vitamins."
These "folks" want you to think vitamins, which are part of the
body and are needed for life as their name states, are dangerous
substances. But, they would like you to take a drug everyday as if
it were a vitamin?! To prevent heart attacks and cardiovascular
disease, we recommend strongly against aspirin. *Instead* take the
cardiovascular nutrients and anti-oxidants outlined in this chapter.
Indeed, aspirin inhibits the synthesis of Vitamin C and interferon.
*In the U.S., in any given year, hundreds of people die or need
hospitalization from aspirin toxicity or allergic reaction.* The number of such incidences from taking the cardiovascular nutrients in
most years is *zero*. Neither will you have an increased likelihood
of a stroke as is the *proven* case with aspirin. Aspirin is very
allergenic and can cause ulcers or other gastrointestinal disease.

ANTI-OXIDANTS
Vitamin A
Vitamin C
Vitamin E
Vitamins B$_{1,2,3,5,6}$
B$_{15}$ (or N,N Dimethylglycine)
Bioflavonoids
Selenium
Glutathione
Cysteine
Zinc
Superoxide Dismutase (SOD)

Anti-oxidant nutrients have also been called *anti-aging* nutrients.
After several decades of *proof* by, (and subsequent persecution of)
medical nutritionists, even mainstream medicine *now* admits that
these crucial nutrients have both anti-aging and anti-cancer properties. It is *highly unlikely* that you will get enough of most, or all, of
them in your diet due to the many factors described at the beginning
of this chapter. Also, as we age, our metabolic processes run down
and we may not absorb or process these nutrients properly.

The anti-oxidants either directly scavenge *free radicals* or they are nutrients that are incorporated into enzymes that perform this task. Recall from the last chapter, that free radicals are *highly reactive* substances and are desperate to attach to anything to get that extra electron. The free radical will thus damage any molecule or cell that it attaches to. Free radical damage ages us. Anything that counters them will enable us to age less quickly and will help prevent cancer too.

Vitamin A is a powerful anti-oxidant and anti-cancer nutrient. It occurs in high amounts in fish liver oil. Its precursor (or pro-vitamin form), beta-carotene, is found in carrots, sweet potatoes, beet greens, broccoli and similar vegetables. The minimum Recommended Daily Allowance (RDA) is 4000 units (I.U.'s) for adults. Most medical nutritionists, however, have long recommended ten to twenty thousand units a day as a preventative measure. In extremely rare cases, much higher daily amounts of the fish oil form of Vitamin A, led to problems. The precursor form, beta-carotene, is much less likely to cause any problems. However, if, as we age, we cannot convert the precursor form to the actual form the body uses, then the fish oil form must be ingested. By eating some fish and the vegetables noted above or drinking occasional carrot juice, you can get some of both forms of Vitamin A. It will also be found in most multivitamin/mineral supplements — as will most of the anti-oxidants and cardiovascular supporting nutrients. Buy your "multi" in a health food store. Avoid the pretty, but artificially, colored supplements made by the drug companies. They also usually contain far less of the various nutrients than do most brands sold in the health food stores.

Vitamin C (ascorbic acid) is a great anti-oxidant, anti-aging nutrient and anti-stress nutrient. Much research on this nutrient's abilities has been performed, for decades, by two-time Nobel Prize winning chemist, Linus Pauling, PhD. The RDA is set at 60 mg. Dr. Pauling recommends a daily dose of 250 mg. to 10,000 mg. as optimum. The need for Vitamin C can be clearly manifested in those that supplement with it. A darker (than usual) urine color may indicate that you've taken more than enough. You can take up to this threshold amount. Under any stress, such as from a cold, a much higher dose would be required to see this color change in the urine. Your body needs more and is using it to fight the germs! Note our nutrient recommendations are geared not merely to keep you from imminent death from scurvy. They are geared to safely maximize your longevity and your health. Most nutritionists recommend 500 to 1,000 mg. as a daily, preventative measure.

Some of the common food sources of Vitamin C, such as citrus fruits, are also very common allergens. We have found that many people do experience bladder frequency, even burning pain on urination and (rarely) stones from a large Vitamin C intake. Here we agree with mainstream, medical physicians and ask that the holistic physicians stop ignoring these common complaints. (You see, being a *physicist*, and *not* being a physician, leaves this author out of *both* "good old boys' clubs" with their own prejudices.) Always remember that taking a vitamin everyday can lead to allergic reactions in many people; just as eating the same foods everyday can.

So there is a dilemma regarding Vitamin C. We need high amounts of this nutrient. But, we must try to avoid negative, or allergic, reactions from citrus fruits or common forms of this supplement. One answer[20] is in the newer Ester-C® form of Vitamin C. It does not cause the bladder frequency complaints. Buy it without added bioflavonoids, if possible. These latter, citrus-derived nutrients also cause much bladder (or other) distress in many people.

Vitamin E helps prevent cardiovascular disease, including heart attacks, and it is a powerful anti-oxidant. Most medical nutritionists recommend at least 100 IU daily, with a gradual build-up to 400 IU daily. Its sources in supplements include wheat (if listed as natural and not declared to have any other source), soy and synthetic derivatives. If you use oils in cooking (which we earlier recommended against) or (better) in salads, you can place some Vitamin E — pop the capsule — in the oil container and keep it in the refrigerator.

The various anti-oxidant, B-Vitamins listed — B_1 (thiamine), B_2 (riboflavin), B_3 (niacin or niacinamide), B_5 (pantothenic acid) and B_6 (pyridoxine) — are also needed by the nervous system, the liver, the immune system, for blood cell formation and for many other purposes. As we age our livers have trouble converting some of these vitamins from their precursor forms to the actual form the body uses. Ask your heath food store for brands that contain Vitamins B_2 and B_6 in the already converted form. Riboflavin (B_2) becomes Riboflavin-5-Phosphate and Pyridoxine (B_6) becomes Pyridoxal-5-Phosphate. So senior citizens, or those with liver disorders, should try to buy a B- complex or multi-vitamin-mineral with some of these two vitamins in the converted (or phosphorylated) forms.

Vitamin B_6 alone is needed for many purposes. It's needed in amino acid metabolism — thus to form hormones, neurotransmitters, enzymes, antibodies, red blood cells, etc. It's needed in fatty acid and carbohydrate metabolism and for cardiovascular metabolism and for proper, neurological functioning. It can reduce edema, help make stomach acid, help Vitamin B_{12} absorption, and can eliminate carpal tunnel syndrome in some people. A decade ago, a study attained much media attention. Six people developed neurological symptoms[21] after daily ingesting thousands of milligrams of Vitamin B_6. We recommend you take a B-complex or multi-vitamin-mineral with about 50 milligrams of these B-Vitamins. (The RDA is of the paltry order of a milligram or so of these B-Vitamins.) But it is not true, as some books by nutritionists seem to indicate, that more is always better.

B_{15} (or N,N Dimethylglycine) is not yet universally recognized as a B-vitamin. This nutrient has tremendous ability to increase the level of oxygen in your tissues. You can get this supplement, as a sublingual, dissolvable tablet, in your health food store.

Supplements of bioflavonoids — in Europe these are called Vitamin P — are usually derived from citrus fruits, which we have said are common allergens. Other food sources include buckwheat, black currant, plums, apricots and rose hips. This class of nutrients

works with Vitamin C. Instead of the potentially, allergenic supplements, we recommend here that you eat the above foods that
contain bioflavonoids. Try to rotate them; don't eat the same one
everyday. That's how you develop a new allergy/addiction.
Selenium is a very powerful anti-oxidant and anti-cancer mineral.
It works with the tri-peptide (three amino acids) glutathione to
detoxify the dangerous lipid peroxide *radicals* found in all heated
oils and in other substances. Selenium is found in high amounts in
fish and seaweed. Selenium also helps counteract the toxic metal,
mercury. The Japanese diet, which is high in seaweed and fish,
contains up to 1000 micrograms of selenium daily. Most medical
nutritionists recommend a daily supplement of 200 micrograms.

By the way, virtually all enlightened physicians strongly recommend that you go to a holistic dentist and have all of your so-called
"silver" amalgam, dental fillings replaced if you really want to live
as long as possible! These amalgams are really more *mercury* than
they are silver. Unbiased studies by Swedish metallurgists proved,
in 1987,[22] that half the mercury leaches out within a few years and
goes into the body. Sweden, Germany and Austria are banning the
use of mercury, dental amlgams. Mercury is one of the most
powerful toxins known to man. It can cause great harm to the
immune system, the nervous system, the kidneys and more.
Replace the amalgam with a porcelain/ceramic composite. But go
only to a holistic dentist who has been doing this replacement for
years. Ingest all your anti-oxidants, in high amounts before your
visit to replace the mercury amalgams. Especially take Vitamins A,
C, E, and selenium and the amino acid cysteine.

Glutathione should be purchased only in the "reduced" form.
Otherwise it will come as the three separate amino acids it com-
prises. But there is no guarantee that your body will combine the
three to make glutathione; so buy the reduced form. Glutathione is
a powerful anti-oxidant. Along with Vitamin C and the amino acid,
taurine, it's being found useful for cataracts. Glutathione is part of
the glutathione peroxidase enzyme that will counteract the
dangerous lipid (fatty) peroxide radicals described above.

The anti-oxidant mineral, zinc is also needed for healing, for the skin and other connective tissue, and for making insulin. As we age, the loss of a sense of smell or taste may be tied to zinc deficiency. Superoxide Dismutase (SOD) counters the superoxide free radical. In August, 1993, a disorder of this anti-oxidant has been found[23] to cause the genetic form of the disease, ALS. ALS (Amyothrophic Lateral Sclerosis), also called Lou Gehrig's Disease, is a neurologically degenerative disease. SOD also has benefit in counteracting radiation-induced tissue damage. It's a naturally occurring enzyme in the body; it can be bought in health food stores.

Finally, as we close this discussion on anti-aging nutrients, a word on some commonly, dispensed bad advice. Some aging "experts" recommend every substance touted for these purposes, including new and potentially dangerous *drugs*. This is equivalent to the American military tactic during the Vietnam War: "In order to save the village, we had to destroy it." Of course, this is nonsense, for your health and longevity, concentrate on *natural* substances, not drugs. The nutrients described here are part of the body, drugs are not.

A NOTE ON ARTHRITIS

If we make it to a very, ripe old age, we will likely, eventually have some arthritic complaints. The first thing to do is to eliminate nightshades (especially tomatoes and tomato sauce) from the diet. If this fails, get complete food allergy testing, and eliminate the appropriate offenders. (In some cases, inhalation of chemicals can cause arthritic complaints too. Hair dressers — who inhale much ammonia and formaldehyde — have a high incidence of arthritis and lupus.)

We strongly advise you to realize how allergic and toxic the drugs used for arthritic people are. Many people adversely react to the gold, penicillamine or other drugs commonly used for arthritics after aspirin is no longer tolerated. These drugs, *and aspirin*, are not well-tolerated precisely because *they are very, allergic substances and arthritis sufferers are really just very, allergic people.*

Certain nutrients counteract arthritic complaints. Zinc and copper forms of Superoxide Dismutase (SOD) can now be purchased. They have been found to be beneficial for arthritics. Vitamin B5, pantothenic acid, can help boost the adrenals and thus fight inflammation. Arthritics are often low in the amino acid, histidine, especially rheumatoid arthritics. Histidine is found in radishes which may be why this family of foods can cause watery eyes, etc. Histidine is also related to sexual functioning. Histidine is low in those who have trouble attaining orgasm. Food for thought? Now I know you may want to get this nutrient!

Manganese, folic acid and the fish oil, Max-EPA® have been found to be beneficial for arthritics. Of course, you know about the need to get enough calcium in your diet or, more likely, through supplementation. Here it has been proven that daily exercise increases calcium absorption. This is crucial if longevity and optimum health are your goals. Good food sources of calcium include, fish, soybeans, almonds and broccoli. We strongly recommend against dairy products.

Furthermore, it is crucial that you take in as much magnesium as calcium. Older nutritional recommendations were to take twice as much calcium as magnesium. This can create a serious magnesium deficiency which can lead to fatigue and viral disorders.

The supplements cited in this chapter can help you live longer and can prevent cancer and cardiovascular disease. It's time for a trip to the heath food store. Pick up some organic produce while you're there.

6

WEIGHT LOSS BREAKTHROUGHS FOR LIVING INTO YOUR 90'S

The two things universally acknowledged to increase longevity are a physically active life (through work or exercise) and being thin. Here we will examine some of our discoveries that can help you lose those excess pounds and keep them off.

For many of us, the standard dogma about limiting calories is not enough or appropriate for us to reach our ideal weight. We will concentrate on novel approaches that include the idea that many people can attain their ideal weight *regardless of caloric intake*. Now, many who can't lose weight by watching calories can be comforted; with the knowledge from this chapter, they should finally have success.

CAUSES OF WEIGHT GAIN AND/OR ADDICTION REVEALED

1. Faulty appestat. The turn on/turn off cells in the Appetite Control Center (appestat) in the hypothalamus in the brain may be malfunctioning from histamine or other substances released from allergic reactions. *Instead of turning off, they turn on, as the allergic food is eaten.* So one gets *hungrier*, not satiated as one eats an offending food. Some people can't stop eating until they run out of the final frontier — space.

2. Disordered water metabolism. This mechanism may even

relate to our Heart Integration™ techniques. Certain food (allergies) are likely keeping water on you. Does your urine vary in density and color? (Of course, men can more easily answer this than women can.) Do you get thirsty after eating certain (non-salty) foods? Assuming no involvement of drugs, vitamins, salt, etc., this is likely due to allergic reactions. Eating allergic foods may cause you to retain water and the urine is darker, more concentrated, and less urination occurs. Some common foods that do this to many people include tomatoes, dairy, vinegar, wheat, and beef.

Here substances, such as histamine, released from allergic reactions, may affect the hypothalamus-pituitary-kidney-heart link that regulates water metabolism and blood pressure. The hypothalamus — which is involved in the body's water metabolism — has been found to contain many histamine receptors.[24] Eating a food that causes this abnormal, but common reaction, causes a false signal that the body is dehydrated. The body will then keep too much water in it as a reaction. Avoiding these (allergic) foods *resets* the water regulation and diuresis (large urinary loss) results with a clear urine demonstrated. But continually eating the offending foods never allows the water "regulators" to re-set.

When the author's allergies were bad, a single tomato could lead to a water retention of several gallons. Avoiding this food then led to a large water (and weight) loss. The author once lost six pounds in an hour! (We have a urine-analysis to prove it. The specific gravity was virtually that of pure water.)

3. Hypoglycemia. This can lead to a craving of sweets or any (allergic) substance that affects blood sugar. If you eat a meal and *then* have to have sweets, some food has dropped your blood sugar; presumably by an allergic response affecting your pancreas. You may then be unable to stop yourself from pigging out on cake, cookies, ice cream or want a shot of caffeine too. The "cure" is to identify which foods cause you to crave the sugars and eliminate these foods.

4. Disordered methionine metabolism.[25] The essential amino acid — methionine — is improperly metabolized in many people. *Toxic,*

addictive, endorphin-like (opium-like) substances may be produced in the body. This may explain why many people *eat only a few foods*. They experience some kind of "high" from these foods. This is from the endorphin effects on the brain. Foods that don't elicit this reaction aren't eaten. But the resulting endorphin-like substances are toxic to the brain, liver, pancreas, etc. A vicious cycle begins. *Learn to eat foods that don't get you high.* Getting high on a food is a sign of the allergic/addictive mechanism and this will cause you to gain weight as well as to experience some symptoms of (hidden) food allergies.

5. Candida-Yeast Syndrome. Do you crave foods that contain both sugar *and* yeast/mold foods? Foods that contain yeast/mold include alcoholic beverages, cheese, dried fruits, mushrooms, anything that contains vinegar (such as mustard, mayonnaise, ketchup, salad dressing preparations, and pickles). Note the classic ice cream and pickles craved by many pregnant women. Pregnancy is when many women first develop a Candida-Yeast infection. But the Candida-Yeast Syndrome also affects many men. Craving things with vinegar is often a give-away here. Learn to avoid these foods. They will cause you to overeat and often will adversely affect your water metabolism too.

6. Exorphins.[26] Certain foods have recently been found to contain exorphins — opium-like substances *already formed in the food*. So *everyone* can potentially get addicted to these foods! It may be *unnatural, and dangerous* to eat any of these foods. Wheat gluten, milk casein and legumes (such as peanuts) are exorphin proteins. Giving up wheat and dairy are often crucial to losing weight. Do you know many people who don't crave these two or the ultimate, addictive food — pizza? Or is it ice cream? (Milk and sugar.)

For the record, wheat is an unnatural hybrid only grown in the last thousand years or so. We've already said that cow's milk was meant for baby cows. Peanuts also contain large amounts of the mold product, aflatoxin which is one of the most potent toxins and carcinogens known to man. So while the foods containing exorphins may make you high, they can lay you low; and they make you overeat and gain weight.

7. Avoiding or minimizing fats. Some people lose weight only when they count *not total* calories, but *fat-containing* calories. These people may have hidden digestive or metabolic problems. (Fats also have twice as many calories, per unit weight, as do carbohydrates.) As always, we seem to crave what's worst for us — due to our body's ability to make endorphins when we start to get sick. Our advanced metabolism prevents us from feeling sick when we might be better off that way. Then we would more easily know what foods are bad for us. If you crave those fats and oils, they're probably bad for you. Many people have sub-clinical, gallbladder problems. If you have a problem with fats, avoid — or at least significantly cut down on — meats, nuts, seeds and dairy products. Don't eat foods processed or cooked with oils. Even your vitamins can be obtained in non-oily form. For example, instead of a Vitamin E (oily) capsule, you can buy the "dry" powder form in better, health food stores.

With our methods, success often occurs *without* having to eat small amounts of food! It might shock those who have fought the weight battle for years, but *if non-allergenic foods are eaten, one feels satiated after very small amounts.* But, that slight "high" from endorphins or exorphins will be missing and may take some getting used to. [See the back of this book for our healing tape which offers quick help for overcoming addictions and staying on your diet.]

To sum up, the previously, unsuccessful dieter needs complete testing for allergies. Food allergies that cause water retention or bingeing must be avoided. Avoid simple carbohydrates — sugars. This will help hypoglycemics. But do eat the complex carbohydrates — they're best anyway. Most people need to avoid dairy, peanut products and wheat as they contain the addictive exorphins. Many others find tomatoes and beef need to be avoided. Watch for changes in the color and amount of your urine to help determine which foods affect your water metabolism. Then you shouldn't need us to tell you what to do about those foods. If you start to crave *new* foods everyday, you should also know what that means. That's right! And *you're* starting to become the expert on allergies — as it should be!

Keep a diary, if you're not sure of what food and psychological factors may cause bingeing or water retention. Learn to be honest with yourself. Anything you crave or eat everyday may be the cause of your weight problems. Do get all the help and support that you need to help you stick to these weight loss breakthroughs.

Pictured on the next page are some before and after photos given to us by two clients. The before photos are not full-body because, as is often the case, some people are too shy (because of their weight) to take such photos.

An interesting thing is that these ladies look years younger in the *"after"* photos than they did in the "before" photos, when they actually *were* years younger! These women lost all excess weight without any calorie counting at all. Their "hidden" allergies, or allergy/addictions, were identified. They then avoided these foods. They found it easy to love the foods that were good for them and to give up their former addictions. They look better because these hidden allergies were also affecting their health, even if it was "subclinical."

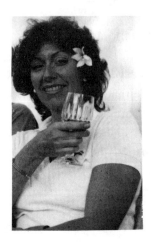
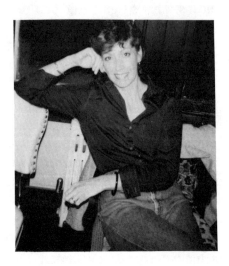

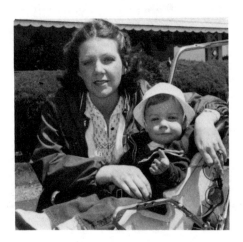
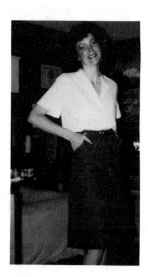

Figures 13 - 16. The first "science of weight loss" results. The "before" pictures are on the left, and the "after" pictures are on the riight.

7

BREAKTHROUGHS FOR RAPIDLY NORMALIZING BLOOD PRESSURE

We have devised two separate, revolutionary, and non-drug ways to rapidly normalize blood pressure. One is to perform any of the three Rochlitz Heart Integration™ Exercises. The other is the dietary elimination of a class of foods containing *monoamines*. If you do not have a diseased heart, kidneys or circulatory system, making both these changes will almost always lead to success. Indeed, either alone may do the job; but the positive effects of Heart Integration™ Exercises may not last if certain foods initiate and re-initiate a high (or in some people a low) blood pressure reaction. If you can attain your goal of normalizing your blood pressure without drugs, isn't it worth making these changes and performing our exercises? High blood pressure drugs and diuretics have many side-effects including gout, depression, impotence and a potentially life-threatening loss of necessary minerals.

CAUTION: If the reader has a disease condition of the heart, kidneys, blood vessels, or related organs, these methods may not work and you should consult your physician first.

Salt and cholesterol in the diet are not the *cause* of most people's high blood pressure. This is another medical myth! (But cutting down on salt and cholesterol is still a good idea.) Though we've seen high blood pressure normalize after people performed our Heart Integration™ Exercises, the dietary factors causing high blood pressure *are* known! The medical profession is not being honest when they say the cause is unknown or "*idiopathic.*" Assuming no cardiovascular or kidney disease, most people could normalize their blood pressure on their own! In the mid-1970's, this author came across some nutrition texts written over thirty years ago. These texts stated that many headaches may be due to foods containing a class of chemicals called monoamines. They are vasoactive — they affect the diameter of blood vessels. (We believe any allergy can do this in susceptible people.)

AVOID FOODS CONTAINING MONOAMINES
CHEESE
YOGHURT
WINE
ANYTHING AGED or FERMENTED
COFFEE
CHOCOLATE
CITRUS FRUITS
BEANS
BANANAS
ANY ALLERGIC REACTION CAN POTENTIALLY AFFECT YOUR BLOOD PRESSURE

Let's start with cheese. It is no coincidence that certain ethnic groups — such as Afro-Americans — have both an intolerance to dairy products and a high incidence of elevated blood pressure. (Unfortunately, as always, if there is an allergy to dairy products, there may also be an addiction.) I have reported these diet changes to people with elevated blood pressure for nearly two decades now and virtually always saw people normalize their own blood pressure within days of eliminating foods containing monoamines especially *cheese* and *yoghurt*. Contrary to its wonderful reputation, we have found yoghurt to be absolutely one of the worst offenders here!

Assuming, again, no pathology (medical disease) exists; we say that "cheese causes high blood pressure most frequently and the *most moldy* cheese — like blue cheese and brie — causes the *most elevated* blood pressure!" This correlation is usually verified at our international lectures when we invite audience feedback. Monoamines are found in anything aged, fermented or malted. This includes alcoholic beverages and anything that contains vinegar. Monoamines are also found in coffee, chocolate, citrus fruits, some beans and bananas. Monoamines have a similar effect on the entire blood pressure in the body that they have when they produce headaches in certain people. But medicine is not interested in this finding! The western, medical establishment, in this century, unfortunately has been corrupted by greed and collusion with the pharmaceutical industry. Only drugs are considered as potential treatments for chronic diseases or conditions.

As a physicist, this author can tell you *that is anything but science.* Science deals with cause and effect whenever possible. Modern, western medicine, however, is only geared towards masking symptoms with drugs; not with finding out the *cause* of the disease! This type of treatment is not only unscientific — though medical people will *simply declare* it to be scientific anyway — it is also fraught with immense danger. This is because of two factors. 1. The actual cause of the disease is simply ignored and thus is *still active* in the body. 2. A new substance — potentially toxic and foreign to the body — has been placed in the body and the body now has to *counteract it* as all drugs have an *LD-50.*[27] LD-50 is the drug industry's own term for the amount of a drug that will be lethal to 50% of those taking it.

Drugs, of course, have their place. But they should usually be the last resort and not the first. Especially whenever safer, less expensive, more natural and *more scientific* methods exist. They usually do! The side-effects of many drugs are often worse than the symptoms they are supposed to be treating.

If you want to make it to your 90's and beyond, you will have to realize the politics and economics of mainstream medicine and take the responsibility to learn non-drug ways towards health whenever possible. And we don't mean to say that natural methods will always be perfectly safe. Indeed, this author's first book, *Allergies and Candida: with the Physicist's Rapid Solution,* was the first to detail how one can become allergic to certain vitamins. That being said, if you don't avoid the foods with monoamines and won't perform our Heart Integration™ Exercises, you may need a diuretic. However, you should know that the following natural substances have diuretic properties. Garlic, a remarkable food, can lower blood pressure, contains selenium and silicon, and has naturally antibiotic properties against fungus, bacteria and viruses. Celery is very high in sodium, yet it has been proven to *lower* blood pressure! This is part of why we state that sodium alone is not the cause of high blood pressure. Rather, the factors you are learning about in this chapter are.

NATURAL DIURETICS
FOODS
Garlic

Parsley

Celery

VITAMINS
Vitamin C

Vitamin B_6

MINERALS
Potassium

HERBS[28]
Uva Ursi

Juniper Berries

Ginger root

Marshmallow root

Cramp Bark

Please consider eating the above foods, avoiding foods with monoamines, and supplementing with the above nutrients. The herbs listed are readily available in your health store alone or in the above combination. Ginger can be eaten fresh or used in cooking.

Let's get back to our Heart Integration™ Exercises. To keep your blood pressure normal, we advise you to perform one of the three Heart Integration™ Exercises, twice a day. If you are so ill that any exercise may jeopardize you, get your physician's permission to do these exercises. Always remember that they will be just as effective if you do them lying in bed! You should easily be able to rotate our pictures here, in your mind, so that you can do them in a horizontal position. Eliminating diuretics, or blood pressure medications should be done gradually and *with your physician's consent — if* you note a normalizing trend in your blood pressure. You should be able to find a physician that will work with you. If not, check your yellow pages or health food store for a nutritionally-oriented one.

Note: You only need to pick one of the following three exercises.

ROCHLITZ HEART INTEGRATION EXERCISE™

1. Do this while humming.
2. It's a cross-crawl variant; use opposite arm and leg. Start out with the right arm as shown in Fig. 17.
3. As best as you comfortably can, hold the elbow up at shoulder height and out to the side with the lower arm (and hand) making a right angle with the upper arm. The hand and forearm are pointing down at the floor. This is the scarecrow starting position.
4. Next rotate at the shoulder (arm and hand as they were). That is, keep the scarecrow, just rotate at the shoulder towards the left side.
5. As the elbow reaches the midline, flick up the forearm towards the horizontal.
6. *Simultaneous* with the right arm flick, bring up the opposite (the left) knee.
7. Then let them both drop down. That is, the arm drops back to the side while the leg drops to the floor.
8. Repeat with the other pair of opposite arm and leg. Be careful not to do this in a homolateral — same-sided — way.
9. After 30 seconds, add the visual circular tracking. Stop the circular tracking if you get dizzy; instead try to look at the eight diagonal end-points.

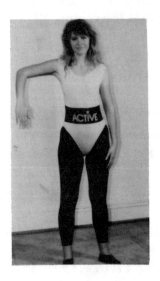 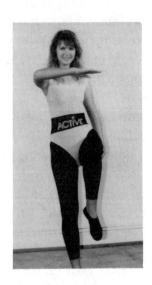

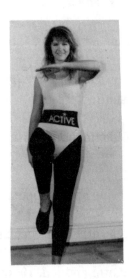 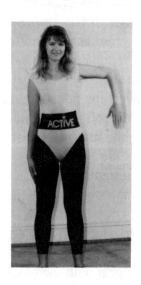

Figure 17 - 20.

Rochlitz Heart Integration Exercise.™ Going clockwise, from the top left:
First half starting position, the first half completed, second half starting
position, the second half completed.

Do the exercise for a minute or two. If you are forbidden to exercise, perhaps the next correction below may be less strenuous. If you are huffing because you don't exercise, maybe it's time to start!

MAESTRO EXERCISE™

1. Do this while humming. (A few will need to count to "switch it on.")
2. With the elbows high and out to the side a bit, trace (with your hands) two "C's" that are back to back.   See Figure 21.
3. Add the circular, visual tracking or track the eight diagonal end-points.

Figure 21.

Maestro
Exercise.™

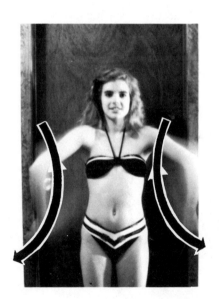

META-MAESTRO™ EXERCISE

1. Do this while humming. (A few will need to count to "switch it on.") See Figures 22 and 23.
2. With the elbows high and out to the side a bit, trace (with your

hands, not your eyes) two "C's" that are back to back.

3. Move your legs in and out to the rhythm of your hands. This is a variation of "jumping jacks." Start with your hands high and feet together. As the hands come down and to the outside, your feet will jump to the outside.

4. Then, the feet will jump back together as the hands go back up and out.

5. Add the circular, visual tracking or track the eight diagonal end-points.

This is usually the most powerful and beneficial of all three Rochlitz Heart Integration™ Exercises.

Do you want to normalize your blood pressure and live into your 90's and beyond? Then please make the diet changes outlined in this chapter, do cut down on the salt intake just to make sure, and perform these remarkable exercises twice a day for at least two minutes each time. The longer you do them, the greater the benefits may be. After all, music conductors often conduct for hours at a time!

Figures 22 and 23.

Meta-Maestro
Exercise.™

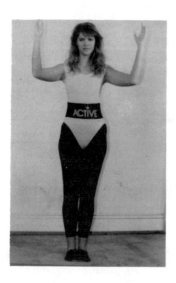 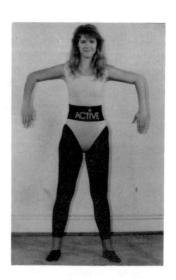

We'd appreciate if enlightened physicians contacted us about doing studies with their patients that they could then send us for publication in a future edition or in the journals. Please: physicians connected to drug companies that manufacture anti-hypertensive drugs need not contact us or pretend to do a "study." Neither should physicians connected to the dairy industry. (We know how *their* results would likely turn out.)

Below, are copies of blood pressure printouts of two students at a seminar in Victoria, B.C., Canada in 1986. Note how their blood pressures went down in minutes. This is truly remarkable because exercising will temporarily *raise* blood pressure. So, likely their blood pressures dropped *even more* than the printouts can demonstrate. An interval of at least a half-hour is recommended before re-taking the blood pressure. But, we had to go on with the seminar. (We have retained the original copies.) The "befores" are on the left; the "afters" are on the right. See also the epilogue for feedback from people who contacted us after their blood pressures normalized from these methods. Please send us *your* feedback on the changes in your blood pressure.

Date: 6/5/86   Date: 6/5/86
Time: 1:06   Time: 1:20
Systolic: 198   Systolic: 161
Diastolic: 123   Diastolic: 104

Date: 6/5/86   Date: 6/5/86
Time: 9:50   Time: 10:05
Systolic: 132   Systolic: 123
Diastolic: 85   Diastolic: 78

8

HAVING A HEALTHY BRAIN INTO YOUR 90'S

In this chapter, we will do for your brain what the Rochlitz Heart Integration™ Exercises have done for your heart and circulation! You are about to enter the fascinating realm of brain hemisphere integration exercises. Spaceyness, poor memory and coordination, difficulty in reading, even dyslexia may have the same lack of brain hemisphere integration as a cause in many cases. Yes, you can be very intelligent and still have a lack of brain hemisphere integration. After examining the simple theory behind this discovery, we'll go over a simple exercise that can correct many of these imbalances! Even sufferers of Parkinson's and Alzheimer's diseases may benefit from performing the techniques of this chapter.

This chapter's recommendations can also rapidly correct dyslexia. So tell your children or grandchildren. Dyslexia means an inability to read. In reality, it is a continuum of reading difficulty with a large percentage of westeners experiencing occasional "mild" forms of reading difficulty. Do you re-read lines, or get sleepy while reading, or can't remember what you read, or have you stopped reading (except for this book, of course)? The "experts" have variously viewed dyslexia as caused by emotional problems, eye or ear disorders and drug deficiencies. They're all off the mark.

Much information on the differences between the left and right halves of the brain has been gained in the last 100 years. Research has been gathered from experiments on people with brain injuries or from those who have had surgical separation of their brain hemispheres. The *left brain hemisphere* is more analytical and temporal; it's in charge of logic, language and mathematical abilities. The *right brain hemisphere* is more emotional, musical, spatial and global.

The two brain hemispheres are joined by the tissue, or set of nerve fibers, known as the *corpus callosum*. It is the corpus callosum, we assert that is not functioning properly in dyslexics and in some of the elderly. Many people nowadays report frequent episodes of falling asleep or tiring while reading, or having to re-read lines. (Many will admit to not reading much. Some may even claim any book they read is too complicated, because they are not yet aware of this problem or too afraid to do something about it.) As we shall see, the *poor memory*, often for *names*, is usually linked to the lack of brain hemisphere integration.

Other signs of this type of problem that we see in the elderly, or others, include the following. Many when asked to touch the left eye, will instead touch the right, or waver indecisively for many seconds. Their personal letters to me often contain transposed letters. Sometimes an "8" is written discontinuously as two little "o's" — one on top of the other. What the faulty "8" may be revealing is that the adult had a brain imbalance as a child — while learning to write. Any difficulty in spinning, car sickness, or trouble riding a merry-go-round may indicate a brain hemisphere integration problem. These learning and spinning problems (early in life) show up long before serious, more (well-known) physical problems ever do.

Now what happens as we read? We read from left to right and when the eyes are left-most in their sockets (the left field of vision), the opposite (that is, the right) brain hemisphere is primarily "activated." Similarly, when looking at the right visual field, the left brain hemisphere is activated. This is an example of the *cross lateralness* of all birds and mammals. You know that the left brain hemisphere controls the right side of the body and vice versa. If a person suffers a stroke in the left brain hemisphere, it is the *right* side of the body that may be paralyzed.

Now the stress of reading — if any — occurs as the eyes move from the left field (right brain hemisphere activated) towards the midline. Before proper control can be transferred to the left brain hemisphere (for viewing the right visual field), the midline is crossed. This activates the corpus callosum. If the corpus callosum isn't functioning properly, problems will then occur. Anything from having to re-read the line to a total inability to read can result. Transposing letters, like "b" for "d" or seeing and writing a backwards "e" are also possible.

The link to *remembering names* in the elderly is clearly a similar type of problem. (We have found this complaint often begins around the age of 40.) Research on those who have had lobotomies or surgical separation of the hemispheres shows that many can see and "know" what an object is when viewed off to the left side, or held by the hand on that side, *but cannot possibly say its name!* Seeing the object in the left field of vision, or holding it in the left hand, activates the right brain hemisphere. The subject can actually see it in his/her "mind's eye." But s/he *can't say it* because the right hemisphere can't get the signal over to the left brain hemisphere where the language functions are! The two hemispheres just can't communicate properly with each other! The different manifestations of reading and other cerebral problems may be due to a continuum of corpus callosum dysfunction. (Note that Orientals, who read vertically, may be spared the stress of horizontal reading.)

Brain hemisphere integration is among the most fragile of energy systems in the body (and thus the hardest to maintain). This is why some super-healthy athletes are known to be dyslexic. Olympic decathlon champion Bruce Jenner and the greatest diver who ever lived, Olympic champion, Greg Luganis are examples. If the dyslexic is otherwise perfectly healthy, like a Bruce Jenner or a Greg Luganis, heart integration™ is undoubtedly maintained. There exists an intrinsic, homeostatic hierarchy in the body. The body, under stress would lose the less survival-oriented mechanisms *first.* Apparently the heart integration™ "circuit" is more crucial than is the brain integration "circuit." You will usually find most who don't have heart integration™ will also not have brain integration and *not* vice versa. *The elderly are the exception.* Many have lost the heart integration™ "circuit."

Now let's return to the fascinating, but simple type of exercise called cross-crawl. Cross-crawling involves simultaneously using the left and right sides of the body. Walking and running properly are cross-crawls. Some aerobic exercises and proper ski technique are also cross-crawls. (See how many have trouble doing them. In the gyms, the cross-country ski machines often lie dormant!) Drs. Doman and Delacato of Pennsylvania were the first to use cross-crawling for those with learning problems or neurological disorders, over 40 years ago. They had people lift up the right arm and left leg simultaneously; then drop them down and pick up the left arm and right leg. This author entered this field in 1983 and devised the following Brain Hemisphere Integration Exercise in 1984.

BRAIN INTEGRATION EXERCISE

1. Start humming. (A small percentage of people may need to count out loud instead. Do it all the way through while humming first. You can always do it through again while counting.)

2. Do a cross-crawl by touching the right hand over to the left knee (as the knee is raised up from the floor). Keep the arm straight (at the elbow) throughout. See Figures 24 and 25.

3. Drop the hand and leg after they touch and then

4. Do the same thing with the left hand and right leg.

5. Repeat this for a minute or two. *It's just like walking in place.*

6. You will sequentially use each pair of opposite arm and leg during this exercise. Do steps 1-6 for a while first before adding step 7.

7. The final step is to slowly, visually track (look at) all the points along a large, imaginary circle in front of you, as you continue the exercise. First gaze along a clockwise direction and then counterclockwise. If you get dizzy, stop and sequentially look at

the eight diagonal end-points.

Figures 24 and 25.
The Brain Integration Exercise. Touch the opposite side of the opposite knee; use both pairs of opposite arm-and-leg. Like walking!!

Left figure: One half—the right arm and left leg combination. Right figure: The left arm and right leg combination.

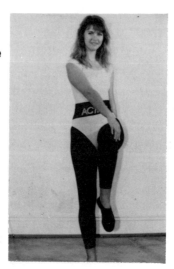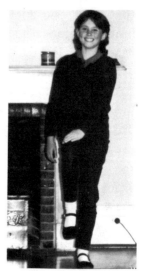

**STOP READING NOW!   PLEASE DO THIS SIMPLE
CORRECTION NOW!**

You may want to use a mirror or have someone watch you, if you are spacey. Wanting to touch the same side arm and leg may be a sign of "dyslexic tendency." This is a desire to perform homolateral (same-sided) crawl as cross-crawl is not yet "switched on."

You can do everything slowly, if you like. Your partner may "trace" the circle with a hand, or pen, while standing in front of you. Keep the head facing straight in front, use only your eyes for the tracking. This visual tracking makes use of the fact that different regions of the brain are activated while the eyes look in different, corresponding regions.

You may want to have the subject read aloud — before and after the correction. You may want to tape this as some people can be close-minded to rapid improvement! This exercise can help alleviate "classical dyslexia" as well as more minor reading and memory problems! (Applied Kinesiologists can employ additional techniques for these problems, as needed.)

Once switched on, cross-crawling is very beneficial. As before, this correction is not "permanent." Do it as often as you can. Some Applied Kinesiologists have seen benefits in people with Parkinson's or Alzheimer's Diseases, but these people will also need nutritional, and other support.

Brain integration exercises are very beneficial for those wishing to be mentally alert well into their 90's. They can be performed twice a day for at least two minutes each time. Longer is usually better. The exercise can be done in bed too, if need be. You may feel clearer and more energetic, coordinated and balanced. Of course, you will likely read more and remember better. You are correcting what applied kinesiologists call *neurological disorganization.*

So how does our Brain Hemisphere Integration Exercise work? The author's theory is that to correct for lack of brain hemisphere integration, we need to *simultaneously* activate the right brain hemisphere and the corpus callosum. This exercise does precisely this. Any cross-crawl activates the corpus callosum. (This is why cross-crawl is difficult for the dyslexic.) Humming activates especially the right brain hemisphere. Recall, applied kinesiology realizes a specific muscle/acupuncture meridian/organ connection. The particular hand motion (touching the opposite knee) utilizes the applied kinesiology muscle — the supraspinatus — which is connected to the brain.[29] Just as the Heart Integration™ Exercises used a muscle — the subscapularis — that is connected to the heart's acupuncture meridian[30] and to the heart itself.

Why is it that in today's world, so many have poor memory (especially for names), reading difficulty, and problems with coordination and spinning? This author has previously linked dyslexia and possibly some of the other problems to the effects of two chemicals. These are *formaldehyde* and *acetaldehyde.* Both belong to a class of chemicals called *aldehydes.* How can these substances cause the problems cited above?

The answer lies in the *Rochlitz Aldehyde Dyslexia Hypothesis* [31] (or *RADH*) formulated in Dec. 1984. This hypothesis states that either, or both, of these aldehydes can adversely affect the corpus callosum. In particular, the connection of this tissue to the right brain hemisphere (or less frequently the left) is interfered with. Kinesiologists use the term "switched off," as do some neurobiologists. Thus the corpus callosum, and especially its connection to the right brain hemisphere (this researcher hypothesizes), is switched off in people with brain hemisphere integration problems by an aldehyde. Both formaldehyde and acetaldehyde are believed to affect the nerve cell receptors for acetylcholine — supposedly the major neurotransmitter in the corpus callosum.

Let's look at the aldehydes in more detail. *Formaldehyde* is fairly well known. It is a ubiquitous, environmental toxin. It's toxic, allergenic, and carcinogenic; and is found in building and insulating materials, wood products, clothing, foam pillows, rugs, cosmetics (now banned in the U.S.) and even in water and milk. It also became infamous after the Arab oil embargo of 1973. A formaldehyde foam was used as an insulation in many homes. Everything from headaches to phlebitis resulted! Formaldehyde is also used to preserve cadavers. Several physicians have told us that allergies and health problems began during their first year in medical school when they worked extensively with cadavers. (Some have even noted that this may be when some physicians-to-be lose their capacity to see the whole picture, as brain hemisphere integration may have been lost.) Formaldehyde is also produced from the artificial sweetener, aspartame.

Aspartame contains the amino acids aspartic acid and phenylalanine and also 10% methanol. Methanol is the "rot-gut" alcohol that killed or blinded people when the usual alcohol (ethanol) was banned during the American Prohibition of the 1920's. It is the methanol that is processed into formaldehyde in the body. Recent research indicates that many people are susceptible to neurological and other symptoms from ingesting aspartame.[32, 33, 34, 35]

Formaldehyde is also produced by the body. It is a metabolic waste product (as in amino acid metabolism) and is hopefully short-lived.

Acetaldehyde (pronounced like acid-al'-da-hide) has several known sources. It is a yeast/fungal waste product. As we age, many will eventually develop a (subclinical) yeast overgrowth. Acetaldehyde is also found in cigarette smoke, smog (including auto exhaust) and alcoholic beverages. It is supposedly far more harmful to the body than is formaldehyde. Many young people have a brain hemisphere integration problem for the following reason. If a pregnant woman has some (possibly unknown) Candida-Yeast problem [see Appendix A], we assert that the fetus may be born with a *life-long* propensity towards dyslexia, hyperactivity or other problem such as car-sickness, allergies, etc. Senior citizens, however, may develop a Candida problem later on in life as the immune system weakens.

The mother's Candida problem may be vaginal or uterine, but *need not be* as acetaldehyde is very volatile and can enter the blood and travel anywhere. Thus, intestinal Candida overgrowth could be the cause. The acetaldehyde could "switch off" brain integration before the fetus/child ever gets a chance. As we have said, "it's no coincidence that the epidemic of dyslexia and hyperactivity in children is occurring simultaneously with the epidemic of vaginal, and other, Candida problems in the mothers of these children!" If the baby is otherwise genetically strong, no other manifestation of illness may result.

One of our 1984 predictions has been verified. Researchers[36, 37] have found that acetaldehyde does indeed cross the placental barrier and causes fetal brain damage. The study was about acetaldehyde in alcoholic beverages. This is why bars must prominently display a sign warning pregnant women not to drink alcoholic beverages. But clearly this would also apply to acetaldehyde in the mother's body which has been produced by Candida overgrowth.

There is also a nutritional connection for these purposes. The anti-aldehyde mineral, molybdenum, may be very beneficial in maintaining your brain hemisphere integration. Molybdenum is picked up by the liver to create enzymes to detoxify aldehydes.[38] Anyone with those brown, "liver" spots should consider taking yeast-free, molybdenum supplements. At least, it should be in your multimineral supplement.

Now the corpus callosum cells, like all brain cells have a high metabolic rate. They therefore need much oxygen and glucose. Undoubtedly, hypoglycemia and low oxygen states can cause the corpus callosum to malfunction.

Recently, pesticides, and chemical solvents have been found to affect learning and memory;[39] formaldehyde was found to be one of these. Avoid rugs, which emit both formaldehyde and pesticides. The same chemicals, especially pesticides, are being linked to Alzheimer's Disease, Parkinson's and other degenerative brain disorders.

9

BREAKTHROUGHS FOR RAPIDLY OVERCOMING CHRONIC FATIGUE

NEW CAUSES OF CHRONIC FATIGUE
Faulty Blood Sugar Levels
Allergies
Candidiasis
Epstein-Barr (or other) Virus
Parasites
Weather Sensitivity
Sleep Disorder
Dumping Syndrome
Hypothalamus Reacting
Magnesium Deficiency
Energy Imbalance
Cranial adjustment needed
Poor Balance

If we live long enough, we may experience chronic fatigue at some point in our lives. The most frequent reason for a visit to a physician's office is known to be fatigue. Part of the reason for this is the remarkably *poor* results most patients will experience — thus necessitating more visits! Likewise, most works written on this subject leave a great deal to be desired. These variously claim that it's primarily emotional, that you should learn to live with it, that you should just keep going to the same type of doctors or keep taking the same drugs or vitamins. *We* realize that drug toxicities and vitamin allergies can actually cause some of these complaints! (Taking supplements with brewer's yeast was the beginning of severe health problems for this author.)

Here we will present our own breakthroughs on chronic fatigue. Yes, we will tell *and* show you what to do about it, too. All along, we presume you have first been checked, by a physician, for any of the many pathological diseases that can cause this general complaint — and that *these have been ruled out.*

Hypoglycemic (low blood sugar) fatigue often occurs as a tiredness or sleepiness in mid-afternoon. Morning tiredness is also frequent here. A spaceyness or giddiness may be experienced too. These people will crave sweets — and often caffeine and maybe nicotine — *which are causing much of their problem!* When the blood glucose level drops too far, or alternatively, goes up and down too quickly, the adrenals over-secrete adrenalin and other hormones. Thus many hypoglycemics also experience anxiety, phobias, feelings of insecurity or of impending doom.

Food (and chemical) allergies can also cause fatigue. There is often an initial experience of a *high* followed by the withdrawal phase of fatigue, depression, headaches or arthritis depending on age and frequency of ingestion. One organ, the hypothalamus in the brain, has many histamine receptors on its cells. If histamine, from an allergic reaction, goes to the hypothalamus, any or all of the following may result: sleep disorder, depression, food cravings, weight gain, and water retention. This is because the hypothalamus regulates these functions. Here, addiction is to foods that do not necessarily contain sweets or yeast and mold. Don't eat foods that get you high, they'll lay you low. We joke at lectures by saying, "Eat all you want of things you don't like." When you leave certain foods out of your diet, it will always be the one(s) you *don't* eliminate that are your worst allergies! Since they will also be your worst addictions, you may try to fool yourself as many people do.

Mold and pollen allergies alone can cause fatigue. This author, as a young child, experienced extreme fatigue from tree pollens during the Spring. Only many years later, when hay fever symptoms joined the fatigue in the Spring did I figure it out. Typically, allergists didn't want to know about it.

Addiction to foods that contain yeast and mold is often the giveaway of a Candida-Yeast problem. These foods include cheese, alcoholic beverages (which are also craved by some hypoglycemics and allergy sufferers), and anything aged or fermented. The latter includes anything with vinegar in it; such as pickles, mustard, mayonnaise, ketchup and salad dressing. Avoid sweets and foods with mold in them.

People who have the Epstein-Barr Virus (and/or other chronic viral disorders including Herpes, Cytomegalovirus, Coxsackie virus and others) may experience a malaise all day long. It is often brought about or worsened by exposure to chemicals. The chemicals are said to cause the virus to replicate en masse. Avoid all air-borne chemicals. The worst are said to be paints, furniture polish, terpenes and tung oils. People with a chronic viral syndrome also have swollen lymph glands, headaches and sleep cycle disorders.

They will benefit, in the long run, if they force themselves to exercise. Build-up slowly. Yes, you may be more tired and achy in the short run. But our long term advice has been verified by a recent medical study.[40] We have always said, "The more tired you are, the more you need to exercise." Lapsing into a TV/couch potato will just let your adrenals waste away. (Watching TV has been found to leave people more depressed in the long run too.[41]) And for all these factors in this chapter, it is *crucial* that caffeine be gone from your life *completely.* We made a breakthrough in discovering that caffeine freezes the adrenal acupuncture meridian in a low state. Swear off the caffeine forever!

These chronic, viral sufferers often benefit greatly from taking magnesium supplements. Here is a case where nutritional advice caused some part of the problem. This is because, for several decades, nutritionists recommended people take supplements with a calcium to magnesium ratio of two to one. *This induced a magnesium deficiency in many people.* This continues today. Many people need to take calcium and magnesium in a one-to-one ratio — the same amounts of each. The excess calcium creates the effective magnesium deficiency. As we age, we certainly have to make sure we get enough calcium for our bones, but if fatigue is a problem for you, you may need to ingest as much magnesium as calcium. Check all you supplements, including your multi-vitamin/mineral and calcium/magnesium supplements.

This researcher has discovered that many people have an un-suspected *weather front sensitivity.*[42] Most people are aware of the scenario of the arthritic who feels the aches in his/her joints, sometimes a day before it actually starts to rain. The cause is usually a dropping barometric pressure (sometimes accompanied by a rise in humidity). But we have found that for every one who experiences arthritic complaints, 5-10 more people experience fatigue and malaise as the weather front passes through. You can keep a diary, correlating your fatigue with changes in barometric pressure, by calling the weather bureau or by tuning in to your radio or TV. An additional possibility here is the large mold increase in the air as humidity begins to rise. People with weather sensitivity often feel good and energetic *only* when the weather is clear and dry with those lovely blue skies up above.

Recommendations here are to go on a low sodium diet as the sodium can lead to excess cerebral edema (brain swelling). Avoid your food allergies; we've found that the grains (like wheat) can cause or exacerbate this problem. Get checked for Candida and parasite problems because these may be involved here too. Some people may wish to move to a desert, such as the American Southwest. But the other changes above may be enough to beat this problem.

A sleep disorder can arise from any or all of the following factors. Viral disorder, food, chemical, or pollen allergy, hypoglycemia, and cranial faults. Getting a cranial adjustment may correct the last complaint. Cranial faults can be corrected by an expert chiropractor or osteopath. The skull is not one bone; it is composed of many plates that move together and apart as we breathe. These plates can easily get "stuck" which can cause various symptoms. Cranial adjustments are very beneficial for M.S. sufferers, dyslexics, stroke victims, headache sufferers, glaucoma sufferers and those with chronic fatigue. Most chiropractors and osteopaths adjust only the spine. Find an expert in cranial adjustment; you can first try the yellow pages ads.

We have revealed *dumping syndrome* as a cause of fatigue. Dumping syndrome occurs when the pyloric valve — between the stomach and small intestine — spasms and opens too wide. The stomach's contents will then spill into the small intestine in a rapid and large volume. This then causes blood to pool there. The final result is a drop of blood volume *to the brain* — the so-called hypovolemic reaction. You may feel tired or faint. Medical texts will claim this as a complaint only in patients who recently had gastrectomy (partial, stomach removal) operations. But we have found that *caffeine, sugar, dairy products* and other allergies can cause this reaction. Avoid these substances and eliminate carbonated beverages as the extra gas pressure can be a contributing factor too. Have you ever felt tired or woosy all over only to have this feeling *vanish* after you belched? This may be another sign of the dumping syndrome which may occur most often in the morning.

In addition to fatigue, do you also have a history of poor balance, poor coordination, inability to spin safely, or trouble riding a merry-go-round or car sickness as a child? These things can actually be fixed, *in minutes,* with some applied kinesiology techniques. The Brain Hemisphere Integration Exercise is one of these helpful techniques. The other techniques are called Pitch, Roll and Yaw corrections. These are beyond the scope of this book. [They can be learned from the author's book, *Allergies and Candida: with the Physicist's Rapid Solution.*] We will depict some applied kinesiology techniques for you to perform at the end of this chapter. This will likely immediately boost your energy level. Again we have presumed throughout that your physician has ruled out a pathological disease in your case.

Finally, we note that mainstream physicians have at last recognized chronic fatigue syndrome. As we predicted, in our first book, they have given it their own names. They call it fibromyalgia or fibromyositis to denote that sufferers often have much muscle fatigue and pain. As always, (experimental) drugs are all they are interested in — never the cause of a disease as science dictates. In fact, mainstream physicians have delineated pain points on the body in fibromyalgia sufferers. They recommend never touching these areas. This turns out to be quite ludicrous, as most of these points are known from applied kinesiology as neurolymphatic points. To make the long story short, many of these people can only recover if they receive stimulation at these points![43]

THREE FACTORS IN DISTINGUISHING CAUSES OF FATIGUE

1. Distinguishing complaints
2. Type(s) of allergy present
3. Types of cravings or addictions

This chapter can help you determine what may be causing your fatigue — the most common complaint of all. Distinguishing complaints (Number 1 above) tells you to look for *non-fatigue* complaints that are specific to each possible factor. For example, the Chronic Epstein-Barr (or other) Virus usually causes swollen lymph nodes, while the other causors probably do not. The type of allergy (Number 2) means to use the allergy/micro-organism link (see below.) The third factor relates the type of foods you are addicted to, with the possible cause(s) of your fatigue. If you have *only* hypoglycemia, your cravings will include sweets (and perhaps some other) allergies. If Candidiasis is present, in addition to sweets, you will crave foods with yeast and mold. Addiction to foods in other categories implies allergies, and that you eat them too often.

TYPE OF ALLERGY — MICRO-ORGANISM LINK

Only Chemical Allergies Implies Viral Disorder
Only Food Allergies Implies Eat Them Too Often
Only Pollen Allergies Implies Candidiasis
Universal Allergies Implies Candidiasis

This list is both simple and remarkable in what it includes. The key factor is the word "only." If you *truly* have *only* chemical allergies and are sure you do not have any pollen or food allergies, a chronic virus may be the cause. Having *only* pollen allergies implies Candidiasis and having *only* food allergies and no chemical or pollen allergies implies that you may be eating those foods too often. Having all types of allergies implies Candidiasis (possibly accompanied by Chronic Epstein-Barr Virus or other virus). This is not a substitute for proper testing.

We are ready now for some applied kinesiology, breakthrough techniques to help you rapidly overcome chronic fatigue. First we'll supercharge your heart and get that blood and nerve energy flowing with the author's Meta-Maestro™ Exercise.

META-MAESTRO™ EXERCISE

1. Start, and continue, humming throughout. (In some cases, people need to count. First do it completely through with the hum. If you feel or see no improvement, go back, and try this while counting out loud.)

2. With the elbows high and out to the side a bit, trace (with your hands) two "C's" that are back to back.

3. Add the circular, visual tracking. If you get dizzy, stop and try viewing the diagonal end-points instead, as you perform this exercise. So far this is just the Maestro Exercise™

4. Now move your legs in and out to the rhythm of your hands. This is a variation of "jumping jacks." Start with your hands high and feet together. As the hands come down and to the outside your feet will jump to the outside.

5. As the hands go back up and towards themselves and then to the outside, the feet will jump back together again.

6. Keep repeating steps 1-5 for two minutes in a continuous fashion. After a short while, this should flow and not be a jerky one step at a time motion.

Figures 26 and 27.

Meta-Maestro
Exercise.™

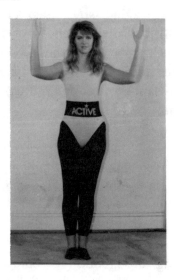 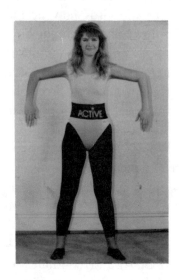

Next we will fire up your "command center" so that your two brain hemispheres work together. This will subtly optimize nerve energy flow throughout your body.

BRAIN INTEGRATION EXERCISE

1. Start humming. (Some people need to count. You can do one then the other as you perform this exercise.) Do a cross-crawl by touching the right hand over to the left knee (as the knee is raised up from the floor). Keep the arm straight (at the elbow) throughout. See Figures 28 and 29.
2. Drop the hand and leg as soon as they touch and then
3. Do the same thing with the left hand and right leg.
4. Repeat this for a minute or two.
5. You will sequentially use each pair of opposite arm and leg during this exercise. Do steps 1-5 for a while first before adding #6.
6. The final step is to slowly, visually track (look at) all the points

Figures 28 and 29.
Brain Integration Exercise. Touch the opposite side of the opposite knee; use both pairs of opposite arm-and-leg. Like walking!!

Left figure: One half—the right arm and left leg combination. Right figure: The left arm and right leg combination.

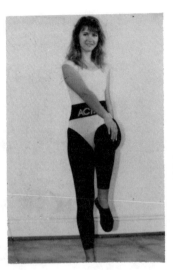
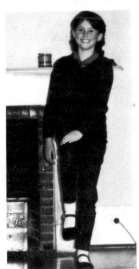

along a large circle in front of you, as you continue the exercise. First gaze along a clockwise direction and then counterclockwise. If you get dizzy, stop and try to view the end-points of the diagonals as you perform this exercise.

Fixing your gait reflexes will wake up those tired legs and you will be amazed at what it will do for your over-all fatigue!

GAIT REFLEXES

1. This correction is a heavy rubbing at the points shown. They are not between the toes, but are a ½ inch or so into the feet. They're between the extensions of the toe bones. Add the bottom of the ball of the foot (not shown.) See Figure 30.

Switching on the ears often improves energy level by a full third. You are also (intrinsically) correcting acupuncture meridian points and chakra (nerve plexus) energies. Your tired or pained neck may also benefit.

Figure 30.

Gait reflex points.
Add the ball of the
foot (not shown).

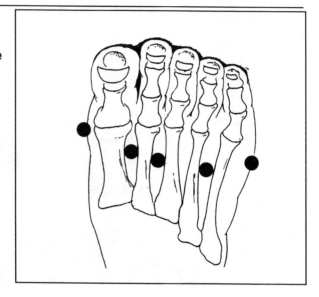

SWITCHING ON THE EARS

1. The correction, see Figure 31, is to *unravel* (radially outward) the outer part of the ear, going completely around (clockwise) as you unravel.

2. Do this five times on both ears.

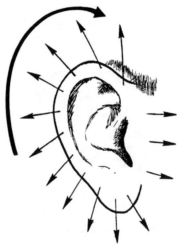

Figure 31.
Switching on the ears.

Finally we have a correction that can help re-set your blood sugar energies through energy balancing. You might be amazed at how quickly you may feel less tired if blood sugar energy imbalance was the cause of your fatigue.

BLOOD SUGAR ENERGY CORRECTION

1. This correction is a two-hand, two-point simultaneous tapping with moderate pressure.
2. One hand will tap one of the two K27 (Kidney 27 acupuncture) points. This point is just under the collar bone and adjacent to the sternum as shown in Figure 32.
3. The other point is the Sp21 (Spleen 21 acupuncture) point. This point is on the side of the ribs as shown. You find it by bending the elbow which is held at the side. Where the inside elbow crease meets the ribs is the Sp21 point.
4. The correction is one hand tapping a Sp21 point and the other hand simultaneously tapping a K27 point.
5. Tap the *left* Sp21 point with the *left* K27 point for 30 seconds. Then tap the *left* Sp21 point with the *right* K27 point. Next, you will tap the *right* Sp21 point with the *right* K27 point. Finally tap the *right* Sp21 point with the *left* K27 point. There are *four* sets of two-hand tappings here.

Figure 32.

"Blood Sugar Energy Correction."

Often helpful for hypoglycemics.

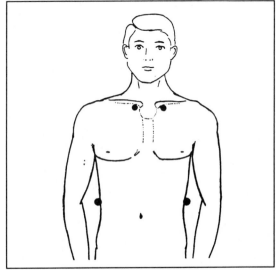

6. Tap each of these four two-point tappings 30 times. You can even tap with a harmonizing waltz beat — HARD-soft-soft.

Send us your feedback on whether, or how, these methods helped you to overcome chronic fatigue.

10

HOW TO INCREASE YOUR STAMINA, STRETCH & ATHLETIC PERFORMANCE IN MINUTES

One of the few universally accepted ways to increase longevity is to exercise vigorously throughout our lives. The groups of peoples, who live very, long lives in various mountain areas — including the Himalayas and the Urals — are known to be very physically active, even *after* their nineties. Of course, just getting about at high altitudes will probably boost cardiovascular performance in a manner similar to exercising. So these people are intrinsically exercising twice as hard as they might be at sea level.

CAUTION: If you're not used to doing any exercise, get your physician's O.K. first.

This chapter is designed to help you boost your athletic performance whether you are an octogenarian (or older), or a 20-year old Olympic Gold medal winner. Bear in mind, that any of our special exercises can even be performed in bed (to supercharge you up), if need be. They can also be performed *before*, *during* and *after* your exercise routine. This is because the energy "switches" they turn on can easily switch off (before, during or after) the exercise regimen.

Before we get into our breakthrough, applied kinesiology techniques, we must remind you of our finding that few things will boost your ability to exercise optimally as much as ascertaining and eliminating your (hidden) food allergies. Allergic reactions usually cause some achiness (in the muscles and joints), and will adversely affect your blood sugars. Some of the achiness may also be caused by an over-acid condition. This can be improved by making the body more alkaline before exercising, by drinking carrot, or celery, or cucumber, juice.

If you find and eliminate your food allergies, you will be able to exercise longer and harder and with less achiness and fatigue. This is analogous to someone who has suffered a car accident. We have observed how some people respond well to applied kinesiology, or chiropractic, or osteopathic adjustments after the accident. Others, however, continue with arthritic-type complaints long after the first group — with similar injuries — has healed completely. This is just another way the body is telling you to get allergy testing.

Some foods to avoid for increasing your athletic performance are universal. Resist the urge to put caffeine in your body. The initial high will later weaken and freeze your adrenals in a low state. (Or in an elevated, nervous state if you are very young.) Avoid all sugar (sucrose) as this will adversely affect your pancreas despite some initial high too. Avoid dairy products and tomatoes to cut down on arthritic complaints. Carefully examine your urge to eat the same foods everyday. These are your likely allergens. Get most of your calories from complex carbohydrates like rice, millet, oats, buck-wheat, potatoes (arthritics check this one out), sweet potatoes, beans and truly fresh seeds and nuts, if you can find these. You've also got enough protein here if you eat the beans and grains. If you are not a vegetarian, add turkey and fish. When you need something very sweet, have fruits — papaya is often the least allergenic, we have found — or carrot juice *already* prepared.

A key to being a life-long athlete is to find some form of exercise that you enjoy. Swimming is one of the least stressful forms of exercise on the body. But many people react to the chlorine used in pools. You can clean the water with less allergenic substances such as bromine, and even better, ozone. Do you like competition? These people may enjoy basketball, racquetball, squash, volleyball, soccer, football, tennis, and even ping pong. (Of course, for these you will depend on others to play with. This is not the case with swimming or running.) If you don't like competition, you can also consider aerobics, with some Nautilus or weight training. The least stressful way of running is to buy an inexpensive mini-trampoline and jog in place. This will be easy on your joints and muscles and can "jog" and unclog your lymph system! If at all possible, we would recommend martial arts, because this form of activity usually includes much stretching, yoga-type activity, meditation, and, of course, self-defense. Yoga and tai-chi are fine too. Yoga will be great for your mind and for stretching those muscles. Indeed, we had a wonderful experience with a long-time yoga practitioner at a seminar in Melbourne, Australia. This lady could never do a full split (stretching the legs all the way out to the sides). She felt badly because all her colleagues who had studied yoga for as long as she had, could easily do this. After she performed the Rochlitz Heart Integration Exercise, ™ she cried tears of joy and of enlightenment as she easily did her first full split!

Find something you will love and want to do for the rest of your life. We have always loved sports. This author has been quite excellent in karate, racquetball, ping pong and *air hockey*. We've also run up to half-marathons and have ventured into tennis and skiing. Walking, running and skiing, we note, are cross-crawl activities and will thus be good for your brain and heart (especially if you *hum* as you go along.) If you use the proper hand motion, as described here, you can even integrate your brain, or heart, hemispheres as you walk or run!

We are ready now for some rapid, applied kinesiology, breakthrough techniques to supercharge you and to rapidly increase your stamina and stretch. We'll first supercharge your heart and get that blood and nerve energy flowing with the author's Meta-Maestro™ Exercise. (Note: the other two Heart Integration Exercises — the Maestro Exercise™ or the Rochlitz Heart Integration™ Exercise — can be used instead. But the Meta Maestro™ Exercise is the most powerful. We've proven that with research on athletes.

It will increase your cardiovascular output more than the others, and just as quickly.)

Perform it before, during, and after your exercise routine. Doing it before will increase your stretch and thus make it less likely that you will injure yourself. This is *not* a substitute for your stretching routine, but an addition. Your endurance will also be increased. If you are just starting to exercise, or are very senior, you should still go slow and work your way up. Slowly increase the parameters of your exercise regimen: time, distance, speed, etc. Perform the Meta-Maestro™ exercise *after* you finish your exercise regime to again relax and stretch the now-contracted muscles and to help you recover from any fatigue.

META-MAESTRO™ EXERCISE

1. Start, and continue, humming throughout. (In some case, people need to count. First do it completely through with the hum. If you feel or see no improvement, go back and try this while counting out loud.)

Figures 33 and 34.

Meta-Maestro
Exercise.™

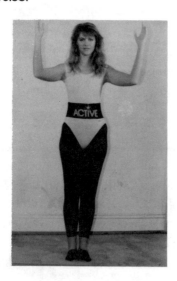 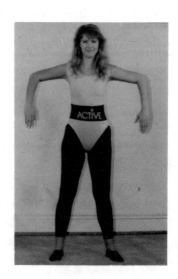

2. With the elbows high and out to the side a bit, trace (with your hands, not your eyes) two "C's" that are back to back.
3. Add the circular (or diagonal), visual tracking. So far this is just the Maestro Exercise.™
4. Now move your legs in and out to the rhythm of your hands. This is a variation of "jumping jacks." Start with your hands high and feet together. As the hands come down and to the outside your feet will jump to the outside.
5. As the hands go back up and towards themselves and then to the outside, the feet will jump back together again.
6. Keep repeating steps 1-5 for two minutes in a continuous fashion. After a short while, this should flow and not be a jerky one step at a time motion.

One type of exercise, we reveal here is somewhat equivalent to the Meta-Maestro™ Exercise! This is jumping rope! The arm motion is "conductor-like" and thus uses the muscle connected to the heart's acupuncture meridian. Since you have to move both feet at the same time, this is somewhat equivalent to our Meta-Maestro Exercise.™

Next we will fire up your "command center" so that your two brain hemispheres will work together. This will subtly, optimize nerve energy flow throughout your body. This one is good to do *before* you exercise.

BRAIN INTEGRATION EXERCISE
1. Start humming. (Some people need to count. You can do one then the other as you perform this exercise.) Do a cross-crawl by touching the right hand over to the left knee (as the knee is raised up from the floor). Keep the arm straight (at the elbow) throughout. See Figures 35 and 36.
2. Drop the hand and leg as soon as they touch and then
3. Do the same thing with the left hand and right leg.
4. Repeat this for a minute or two.
5. You will sequentially use each pair of opposite arm and leg

during this exercise. Do steps 1-5 for a while first before adding number 6.

6. The final step is to slowly, visually track (look at) all the points along a large circle in front of you, as you continue the exercise. First gaze along a clockwise direction and then counterclockwise.

Figures 35 and 36.

Brain Integration Exercise. Touch the opposite side of the opposite knee; use both pairs of opposite arm-and-leg. (Like walking.)

Left figure: One half—the right arm and left leg combination. Right figure: The left arm and right leg combination.

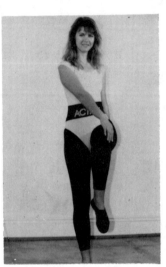
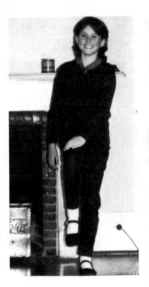

Fixing your gait reflexes — see Figure 37 — will wake up those tired legs and you will be amazed at what it will do for your over-all fatigue! This is a remarkable technique; you may not realize that your leg reflexes have been switched off (possibly for a long time) until you walk around after someone does this on you! You can, of course, do it on yourself. But, somehow it works best when some-one else puts that energy into you. You'll feel it. Unfortunately, as with tickling, you will feel it more when someone else does it to you. If it hurts, just take deep breaths and imagine you're some-where else. You can do this before, during and after any exercise that stresses your legs. This includes martial arts, gymnastics, walking, running, aerobics, skiing, skating, racquet sports, soccer, football, basketball, baseball, etc. All the techniques in this chapter can even help you recover from minor strains and sprains much more rapidly. Any serious injuries should, of course, be seen by the appropriate expert.

GAIT REFLEXES

1. This correction is a heavy rubbing at the points shown. They are not between the toes, but are a half inch or so into the feet themselves. They're between the extensions of the toe bones. Add the bottom of the ball of the foot (not shown.) Rub for at least 10 seconds on each spot.

If your exercise involves your hands or arms, you will benefit greatly by the following correction. We call it the "hand gaits." Its analogous to the gait reflexes for the legs. You'll need to rub these hand gaits points, if your activity includes the following: boxing, karate, gymnastics, tennis, racquetball, squash, rowing, archery, volleyball, paddleball, handball, ping pong, golf, weight training, and yes — air hockey. These sports all have stressful vibrations traveling up the arm just as running, etc. does with the legs.

Figure 37.

Gait reflex points. Add the ball of the foot (not shown).

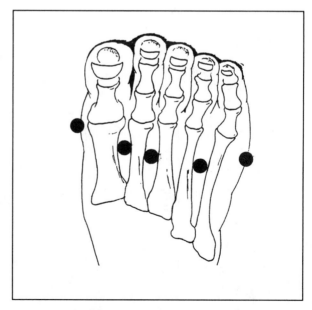

"HAND GAIT" REFLEXES

1. This correction is a heavy rubbing at the points shown. They are not between the knuckles, but are a half inch or so into the hands (in the direction towards the elbow). They're between the extensions of the finger bones. Add the bottom of the "ball" of the hand (not shown.) See Figure 38.

Yes, as its name implies, this correction will better enable you to walk on your hands!

All you Olympic, *and* Sunday afternoon, exercise enthusiasts are invited to send us your feedback after you have used the remarkable innovations in this chapter. Remember, life-long exercise will increase your longevity, release stress, unclog your lymph (detoxifying) system, improve your concentration, optimize your adrenals, and can even balance your emotions. Find an activity you enjoy, learn it, get any necessary equipment and a medical check-up if needed, perform the techniques in this chapter and get going. Yes, into your nineties and beyond as those vigorous people in the Himalayan and the Ural mountains do.

Figure 38.

Hand Gait reflex points.
Add the "ball" of the hand (not shown).

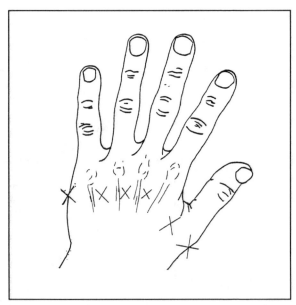

11

BREAKTHROUGHS FOR MULTIPLE SCLEROSIS

The discoveries in this book can help people who suffer from Multiple Sclerosis (M.S.) In this degenerative, neurological illness, the fatty, myelin sheaths surrounding certain nerve cells erode. Limb paralysis, bladder incontinence and eye problems are common symptoms. We include a discussion of this disease here because our discovery of Heart Integration™ Exercises has proven to be one of the most beneficial techniques that an M.S. sufferer can undergo. We cannot promise or guarantee great results for all M.S. sufferers. The least benefits usually occur for those who have had all four limbs seriously affected for many years. But even these people may experience some benefit, but it may take much longer to see any changes. We have observed the greatest benefits for those that have had neurological deficits on only one side of the body or those who have one side much worse than the other side. (Or those that recently developed the problem.) Indeed, the very first subject the author had, after devising the Rochlitz Heart Integration™ Exercise in 1985, was an M.S. sufferer. This woman had a bad limp and a loss of sensation in one foot, for 15 years. After performing our Exercise, she got sensation back in the foot in *seconds*. She then ran! A virtually, normal run. Her ankle also unswelled before us in seconds! We believe our Heart Integration™ Exercise apparently gets both blood and nerve "energy" flowing to the whole body. Both circulation and neurological functioning often immediately improve.

We will show you how to use the Heart Integration Exercises™ for those who may be partially or completely paralyzed. Before we go over our special Exercises, let us describe our findings and recommendations concerning M.S. sufferers. These people have many, many imbalances. They are often led down a false path and their bodies are further stressed by taking *experimental,* immuno-suppressive drugs. This will likely be banned eventually. These people also have many allergies and should get complete testing. Most will have allergies to foods, chemicals, pollens, germs (including bacteria) and pets.

Many can trace the start of their worst complaints to a time when they were around cats. Cats contain many dangerous germs which can be contacted from their saliva, nails and hair. Cats contain Candida (yeast), and parasites including the protozoan responsible for the disease, Toxoplasmosis. Researchers have recently found the cause of "cat scratch fever." This is a sweaty, achy condition that some people get when a cat scratches them. Six thousand people a year report this condition and many also report fever, swollen lymph glands, anorexia, and general malaise. These complaints can last several months. The causative *bacterium* is called Afpia felis[44] and is very virulent. Recent research may also have revealed a possible cause of cat allergy. The cat allergen, called Fel dl, coats cats' skins and may have the power to alter the immune system!

We have seen people who started suffering from M.S. merely after moving to a place that had had a cat. Of course, there may be many steps necessary for the final breakdown to have occurred. Many of these people had dogs as children. Some British researchers claim to have found a link to a virus in dogs. We also believe some environmental pollen may be at work in M.S., as the geographical areas where M.S. is high may be linked to tree pollens. Some M.S. sufferers have also reported recovery when they eliminated wheat, dairy or sulfite preservatives (sometimes used on green vegetables and potato products). Others have been successfully treated with desensitization injections of bacterial antigens. Still others have reported success with bee, or snake, venom injections. (We trust some accurate allergy testing is done beforehand.) Speaking only for myself, taking experimental, immune-suppressing drugs is the last thing I would do. Indeed, I was losing sensation in my arms and legs years ago. I got a diagnosis of M.S. Fortunately, I traced it to the phenol preservatives used in the allergy injections I was getting from an allergist. I stopped all these shots and fully recovered. As a scientist, I knew that I should try to find the *cause*. Many M.S. sufferers also have dental amalgam problems. If gold and mercury (deliberately mis-named "silver") amalgams are adjacent to each other, the mercury leaches out much faster than it otherwise would. Holistic physicians strongly recommend amalgam removal and replacement for M.S. sufferers. They recommend you see a holistic dentist about getting porcelain/ceramic composites for the new fillings.

M.S. sufferers also have many cranial faults and need to see an expert chiropractor or osteopath who can perform advanced cranial adjustments. (This was discussed in the chapter on chronic fatigue.)

FOR THE M.S. SUBJECT: YOU MAY NEED UP TO FOUR ASSISTANTS.

In performing our Heart Integration™ Exercises, you may need two to four assistants if the subject cannot move his/her limbs. If the subject cannot stand, have the subject lie on the floor (or on a safe table) with the assistants on their knees (or standing) around him/her. Each assistant is needed to move an arm or a leg in unison with the other assistant(s). Have a "normal" person perform any of the three Rochlitz Heart Integration™ Exercises depicted in this chapter. Once s/he understands it, it should be easy to assign an arm or a leg to a volunteer to use if the subject cannot move it (well enough) him/herself. Have the assistants duplicate the appropriate limb motion precisely and *simultaneously* as called for. They will pick up and move the subject's limbs, if the subject can't. The subject should try to hum (count in some cases) him/herself while the limbs are used in these corrections. This should be done for several minutes twice a day (unless a problem arises) as a minimum. See if the subject feels any differences each time, especially the first time. Test leg abduction, neurological reflexes, etc. In all the corrections below, the subject does the humming (or counting) unless s/he is a mute, in which case good, classical music may be used to "bathe" the subject during the Exercises.

The Maestro Exercise™ is the easiest of the three Heart Integration™ Exercises described here. You need, at most, two assistants here. Of course, if the M.S. subject can at all perform these exercises on his/her own — even if a bit sloppily — this is preferred!

MAESTRO EXERCISE™

1. Subject starts humming. This assumes the subject's left side (arm, leg, or eye) is worse. If the subject's right side is worse, try the counting instead of the humming.
2. With the elbows high and out to the side a bit, trace (with your hands, not your eyes) two "C's" that are back to back.
3. Add the circular, visual tracking or track the eight diagonal end-points. (Unless dizziness or other complaints result.)

Figure 39.

The Maestro
Exercise.™

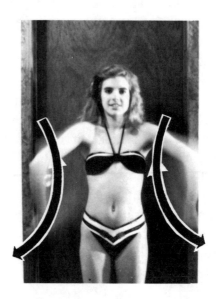

If the legs are not involved in the subject's M.S., the next correction may be preferable. But there is no way to be sure. It is fine and appropriate to try all three heart corrections here — not at the same sitting, if it is too stressful for the M.S. sufferer.

ROCHLITZ HEART INTEGRATION™ EXERCISE

1. Four assistants are preferable here; though it is possible for two people if they are fast and accurate enough. Of course, if the M.S. subject can, at all, perform these exercises on his/her own — even if a bit sloppily — this may be preferred.
2. Subject starts humming. This assumes the subject's left side (arm, leg, or eye) is worse. If the subject's right side is worse, try the counting instead of the humming.
3. This is a cross-crawl variant; use the subject's opposite arm and leg. Start out with the right arm as shown in Figure 40.
4. As best as you comfortably can, hold the elbow up at shoulder height and out to the side with the lower arm (and hand) making a right angle with the upper arm. I.e., the hand and forearm are pointing down at the floor. This is the "scarecrow" starting position.
5. Next rotate at the shoulder (arm and hand as they were). That is, keep the scarecrow, just rotate at the shoulder towards the left side.
6. As the elbow reaches the midline, flick up the forearm towards the horizontal.
7. At this exact time, bring up the opposite (left) knee.
8. Then let them both drop down. I.e., the arm drops back to the side while the leg drops to the floor.
9. Repeat with the other pair of opposite arm and leg. Be careful not to do this in a homolateral (same-sided way.
10. Add the visual circular tracking (after 30 seconds).

META-MAESTRO™ EXERCISE

1. You need four assistants here if the subject cannot use his/her own limbs. This is the most difficult — entails correcting the greatest neurological disorganization — and is therefore potentially

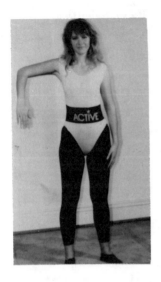 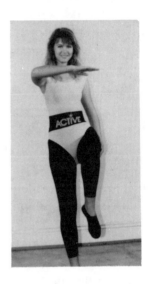

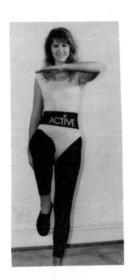 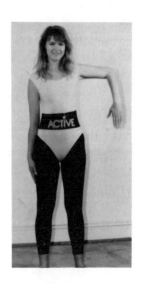

Figures 40 - Figure 43

Rochlitz Heart Integration Exercise.™ Going clockwise, from the top left: First half starting position, the first half completed, second half starting position, the second half completed.

the most beneficial.

2. Subject starts humming. This assumes the subject's left side (arm, leg, or eye) is worse. If the subject's right side is worse, try the counting instead of the humming.

3. With the elbows high and out to the side a bit, trace (with your hands, not your eyes) two "C's" that are back to back.

4. Move your legs in and out to the rhythm of your hands. This is a variation of "jumping jacks." Start with your hands high and feet together. As the hands come down and to the outside, your feet will jump to the outside. Then, as the hands go back up and out, the feet will jump back together. Repeat steps 2-4, continually.

5. The final step is to slowly, visually track (look at) all the points along a large circle in front of you, as you continue the exercise. First gaze along a clockwise direction and then counterclockwise. If you get dizzy, stop and track the diagonal end-points, if possible.

Figures 44 and 45.

Meta-Maestro
Exercise.™

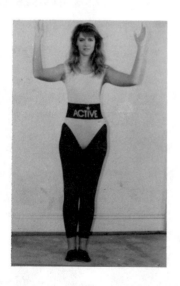 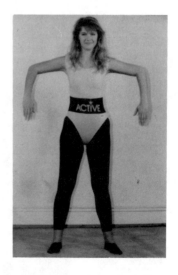

The M.S. subject will also likely benefit greatly from performing our Brain Integration Exercise — especially if there is one side worse than the other — twice a day for two minutes each time (as a minimum). Whenever Heart Integration™ Exercises are performed, make sure the Brain Integration Exercise is done either before or after. For the very first time, we think the Heart Integration™ Exercise should be performed first as listed in this chapter. After that, the order may not be crucial.

BRAIN INTEGRATION EXERCISE

1. You may need two to four assistants here.
2. Start humming (or counting if the right side is worse). Do a cross-crawl by touching the right hand over to the left knee (as the knee is raised up from the floor.) Keep the arm straight (at the elbow) throughout. See Figures 46 and 47.
3. Drop the hand and leg as soon as they touch and then
4. Do the same thing with the left hand and right leg.
5. Repeat this for a minute or two.
6. You will sequentially use each pair of opposite arm and leg during this exercise. Do steps 1-5 for a while first before adding #7
7. The final step is to slowly, visually track (look at) all the points

Figures 46 and 47.
H.E.B.S. Brain Integration Exercise. Touch the opposite side of the opposite knee; use both pairs of opposite arm-and-leg. Like walking!!

Left figure: One half—the right arm and left leg combination.
Right figure: The left arm and right leg combination.

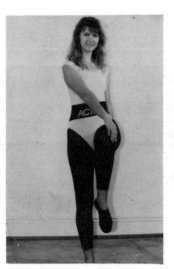
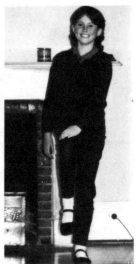

along a large circle in front of you, as you continue the exercise. First gaze along a clockwise direction and then counterclockwise. If you get dizzy, stop and track the diagonal end-points, if possible.

Applied Kinesiologists have discovered a remarkable, reflex system — based on acupuncture — in the feet that may help return some energy flow to the entire leg. Perform this technique on both feet regardless of symptoms. Start out with small pressure, then build-up. Rub each point for 15 seconds.

GAIT REFLEXES

1. The correction is a heavy rubbing at each point. This includes the bottom of the ball of the foot (not shown.)

Figure 48.

Gait reflex points. Add the ball of the foot (not shown).

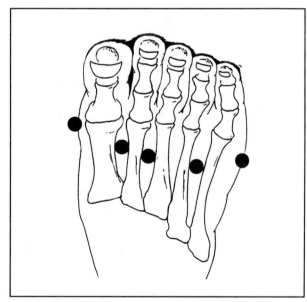

Analogous to the feet points, we have found there are "hand gait" points on the hand that need the same rubbing correction. (Correcting the hand gait reflexes may — together with taking Vitamin B_6 — help overcome carpal tunnel syndrome without needing surgery.) An assistant could perform this technique on both hands.

Start out with small pressure, then build-up slowly. Rub each point for 15 seconds.

Figure 49.

Hand gait points. Add the "ball" of the hand (not shown).

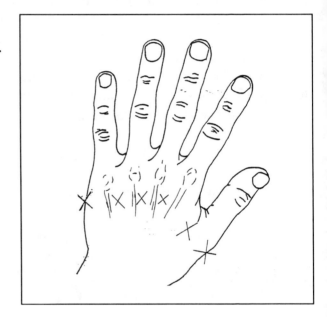

"HAND GAIT" REFLEXES

1. The correction is a heavy rubbing at each point. This includes the bottom of the "ball of the hand" (not drawn.)

When someone is said to be "switched" or neurologically disorganized, it means that their nerve or acupuncture energies are not running 100% in the manner that they should. There may be a confusion between the left and right sides of the body, or the top and bottom, or the front and back. Many complaints can result — from poor balance to dyslexia to chronic fatigue or poor athletic performance. The corrections below should help the M.S. sufferer. An assistant can perform them the first time on the subject. These points should not hurt quite as much as the gait points. Although many people have sensitive K 27 points. (See below.) This relates to a neurological confusion between the left and right sides.

UNSWITCHING

(1) Rub the navel and the two points above the upper lip and below the lower lip as in Figure 50. This helps correct a top/bottom confusion in the body.

(2) Rub the navel and the two K27 points. See Figure 50. The K (or kidney) 27 points are (acupuncture meridian) points under the collar bone, adjacent to the sternum. (The latter is the bone running down the center, to which the ribs attach.) Some kinesiologists say the K27 points must be rubbed daily *until* they no longer hurt.

(3) Rub the navel and the coccyx (tailbone, not shown) which is just above the anus. This helps correct a front/back confusion.

Rub (hard) each set of two-hand corrections for 10 seconds. These three corrections temporarily correct top-bottom, left-right, and front-back switching, respectively.

  Let us know of your results with M.S. subjects. Don't forget all the other recommendations made at the outset of this chapter.

Figure 50.

Unswitching Points. Rub these points while holding the navel. Also add the coccyx point (not shown).

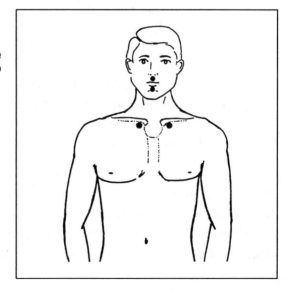

12

EPILOGUE

W e are fortunate to have had people write us of their positive experiences after performing the Rochlitz Heart Integration Exercises,™ in the last few years. Some of this feedback was originally printed in the quarterly journal, *The Human Ecology & Energy Balancing Scientist* (ISSN: 1045-2729). [See the back pages for re-print or subscription information.]

First, we list some of the benefits of performing our Heart Integration™ Exercises. Of course, we hope you will live much longer after your continual performance of the Rochlitz Heart Integration Exercises™! *Let us know in several decades!*

BENEFITS OF HEART INTEGRATION™ EXERCISES
Alleviate Cold hands and Feet
Eliminate *Minor* Cardiac Arrhythmia
Increase Stretch in a Dancer
Eliminate Bruising
Make it Easier to Draw Blood In Children
Lower High Blood Pressure
Get Off Blood Pressure Drugs (With Physician's Approval)
Shorten Labor Time During Childbirth
Overcome The Stress Of Varicose Veins

The Maestro Exercise™ & Giving Blood[45]
Carolyn Thompson, of Smithtown, N.Y. writes, "Recently my eight-year old son was ill and had to have a blood test. The lab technician had great difficulty finding a vein; and after several attempts at drawing blood, was able to extract only a very small

amount. I was told that blood was difficult to draw from children because their little veins collapse easily. This was a very unpleasant experience for my son. You can imagine his feeling two weeks later when I told him he had to have additional blood tests. The bruises had just barely healed from the first attempts. I relayed our difficulty to Prof. Rochlitz, and on his suggestion tried the Maestro Heart Integration™ Exercise just before the next lab visit. *The result was impressive.* A vein was found very quickly, and four vials of blood were filled in just a few minutes. My son was pleased, and he felt more in control of the situation instead of feeling like a victim. The same routine was followed at a subsequent visit with the same successful results. The lab technicians were very interested in my son's exercise, and he taught the Rochlitz Heart Integration™ Exercise to them!"

After Heart Integration, Physician Wonders — Is This Two Different People?
Caution: Consult your physician about cardiac arrhythmias.

Dotty Salinsky of Frackville, PA, writes of her results[46] after performing the Rochlitz Heart Integration™ Exercise. "I went to [a Medically supervised diet/weight loss] Center in Pottsville, PA. Before starting the program, I had to take a physical exam and EKG. After the EKG, but two days prior to the physical exam, my sister Kathryn had me perform the Rochlitz Heart Integration™ Exercises. At the exam, the doctor listened to my heart and looked at the EKG and said, "It seems like two different people, they don't match up; there's no arrhythmia now." He couldn't understand it."

Kitty Kopey writes, "My sister-in-law, Pauline Searles was taking Inderal® for cardiac arrhythmias. She still experienced severe palpitations, and had thoughts of dying. She couldn't sleep well and couldn't remember anything. I showed her how to do the Rochlitz Heart Integration Exercises.™ A short while later, she no longer had any arrhythmia, her memory and sleep greatly improved. During this time, she gradually weaned herself off the drug. After four years, none of these complaints have come back, and she hasn't been taking any drugs."

Rochlitz Heart Integration™ Warms Up Cold Hand[47]

John Cosgrove of Ormond Beach, FL writes, "We have a friend named George who has had a circulatory problem for the past five years. His right hand always seemed colder than his left and would at times seem numb. He tried everything from medical drugs to massage, colonics, and oral chelation to no avail. After studying your Heart Integration,™ he performed the Rochlitz Heart Integration™ Exercise. Within ten minutes, he reported equal warmth in his right and left hands. This corrected condition remains after one month."

Blood Pressure Normalized With Rochlitz Heart Integration™

Janet Mater, R.N. of Ontario, Canada, a graduate of the Human Ecology Balancing Sciences Seminars reports[48] that the Rochlitz Heart Integration™ Exercise has lowered the blood pressure of a hypertensive patient. She says, "We have a 49 year old, overweight lady with moderate hypertension — **160/94** on Dyazide®. After one week of performing the Rochlitz Heart Integration™ Exercise, *she is off Dyazide®* and her blood pressure is 150/88. She performed this exercise while lying down during this first week. After three months of doing this correction, her blood pressure is now **142/82**."

Betty Gilliland writes,[49] "I watched you at a 1986 Health Conference performing your Heart Integration™ and Meridian Integration™ Exercises. In January, 1987, I gave blood and my blood pressure was **130/88**. Since then, I have performed Rochlitz' Heart Integration™ Exercise about a half dozen times. I have also begun to use it with my clients. The great news is that when I gave blood today, my blood pressure was down to **100/70**! Isn't that exciting?! Especially since my family is filled with hypertension problems. I am also going to take responsibility and make the diet changes you suggested, knowing the weight will also drop."

Margaret Hewes, R.N. of Baldwinsville, NY has sent us a preliminary clinical study showing that the Rochlitz Heart Integration™ Exercise normalized high blood pressure in five patients.

Rochlitz Heart Integration Exercise™ Helps Prevent Long-term Injury

Ann Cain of Mullica Hill, New Jersey writes,[50] "I work with animals applying the Rochlitz methods and energy balancing. In January, 1987, I had what might have been a serious accident. I was bashed in the head by one of my horses. Seconds later, while still reeling from the blow, I did the Rochlitz Heart Integration™ Exercise. All bruising and tissue damage was eliminated by the Exercise!! Not a serious blow you say... Well let's talk about the structural work that was necessary. The plates were jammed behind and above the right eye requiring cranial work, the TMJ (jaw joint) was messed up so that the teeth were no longer aligned and the neck and spine required attention.

Recently, my 82 year-old mother banged her shin against the edge of her bed. When she hobbled into the kitchen, I suggested she do the Rochlitz' Heart Integration™ Exercise. She did and guess what? No further pain, tissue damage or bruising of any kind!"

Rochlitz' Heart Integration™ On TV

In Nov. 1987, on the TV show, *A Current Affair*, the 1200 pound man, Walter Hudson, was seen performing a Heart Integration™ Exercise created by Rochlitz — the Maestro Exercise.™ Dick Gregory was interviewed and spoke about the Heart Integration™ theory, which was created by Rochlitz.

Heart Integration Cuts Down On Labor During Birth

Ellen Whooley of Sag Harbor, NY informs us that after attending the BASIC H.E.B.S. Seminar, she performed the Maestro Exercise™ when she thought her labor had begun. Before her physician could rush out and change his clothes, the baby was on her way out. Her entire labor consisted of 1½ contractions — perhaps a record!

Send us your feedback. Physicians: send us your studies. Thanks!

APPENDIX A

ALLERGIES, BLOOD SUGAR PROBLEMS & CANDIDA-YEAST SYNDROME

With increased longevity, you may likely, eventually experience numerous complaints that are due to allergies, blood sugar problems or Candida-yeast syndrome. So we need to examine these chronic problems in detail. We need to learn what causes these syndromes, what symptoms are involved and what to do about them.

Regardless of the complaint, ancient Greek physicians often took their patients off milk, and failing this, *all food* until they got well! While ignored today by most mainstream, medical physicians, allergies cause much chronic, degenerative physical, and "emotional," illness. Allergist, Richard Mackarness, M.D. has stated that allergy is now the prime cause of most medical complaints.[51]

Any harmful effect on the body, brought about by a food, chemical, pollen or energy (such as microwaves, fluorescent lights, T.V., etc.) will be called allergy here. We refer to individual responses. What maladies can allergy cause or be associated with? The following is a partial list. (There are other causes for many of these complaints.)

POSSIBLE ALLERGY SYMPTOMS
Fatigue, dizziness, confusion, headache, migraines, narcolepsy, neck ache, backache, arthritis, gastrointestinal symptoms: gas,

pain, bloating, diarrhea, constipation, esophagitis, colitis, ileitis, hemorrhoids, mouth sores, ulcers, indigestion, repeating a taste, muscle aches and twitches (muscles around your eyes twitch?), double vision, blood sugar problems, rashes, hives and other skin disorders, dermographia (skin turns red or white after slight pressure), bladder frequency, bed wetting, pain on urination, depression, anxiety, paranoia, schizophrenia, cardiac arrhythmias, rapid heart beat, joint swelling, sinusitis, nose runs after eating, shiners under the eyes, earaches, pancreatitis, gallbladder-type pain, high or low blood pressure, anaphylaxis, hot flashes, morning sickness in pregnancy, insomnia, under- and overweight.

When mainstream physicians ask how allergy can cause so much chronic, degenerative illness, we are amazed. After all, if allergy can cause something as "mild" as hay fever and something as extreme as anaphylactic shock (and death), isn't it logical to assume that chronic, degenerative illness which lies between these two extremes can be allergy-induced?! Or would they have us believe that "drug deficiencies" cause all illness?

FACTORS THAT CAN CAUSE ALLERGY

1. Eating the same foods too often. Likewise for overexposure to pollens and chemicals.
2. Genetic predisposition. Many families have members with the same allergic response to the same food.
3. Candida-Yeast Syndrome. Especially if multiple pollen allergies, or "universal" food, chemical, and pollen allergies are present.
4. Lack of breast feeding of infants. Nutrients and protective antibodies not found in any "formula" exist in mother's milk. An entire generation of people have weak immune systems because they did not receive mother's milk. Why? Because Western pediatricians, under the false guise of science, discouraged it!
5. Other organisms or infections can stress the immune system, such as parasites, viruses, etc.
6. Eating toxic, artificial, nutrient-deficient food.
7. Specific nutritional deficiencies especially the anti-oxidants

needed by the immune system.

8. Heavy metal toxicity such as mercury.

9. Fluoride weakens the immune system.

All these things can lead to an immune system breakdown. Allergies, autoimmune disease (like lupus), cancer or immunodeficiency can result. It appears that most people with universal allergies do not get cancer.

HYPOGLYCEMIA & DIABETES — THE ALLERGY CONNECTION

Perhaps the first (often undiagnosed), allergy symptom for many people is faulty blood sugar. William Philpott, M.D., and his biochemist collaborators, have found that the *pancreas* is often directly affected by undigested proteins and fats. Such an organ is called a *shock organ.*[52, 53] Different, undigested foods may preferentially attack different organs or tissues. Wheat gluten, can affect the gastrointestinal tract, nervous system and liver. Philpott has linked allergies with hypoglycemia and diabetes by viewing the pancreas as a shock organ. Causative (allergic) foods need not contain sugar or carbohydrates to shock the pancreas into a high (diabetic) or low (hypoglycemic) blood sugar reaction! This isn't surprising, as many in holistic health know the scenario of the skinny, nervous hypoglycemic who eventually becomes the overweight, fatigued "maturity onset" diabetic.

Hypoglycemia's possible symptoms are listed below.

HALLMARKS OF HYPOGLYCEMIA

(Diabetic — high blood sugar reactions — can also be associated with some of these complaints.) Fatigue, spaceyness, giddiness, mental confusion, sleepiness, frequent hunger pains — even shortly after eating, anxiety, nervous overreactivity, trepidations, insecurity, panic attacks, phobias, depression, muscle cramps, eye symptoms: inability to focus eyes (convergence insufficiency), seeing spots (floaters).

Dropping blood sugar levels alert the adrenals to secrete its hormones. These include adrenalin and other stress hormones. But while running on adrenalin (instead of a steady glucose level) may prevent fainting — it can be a nightmarish existence. The excess adrenal hormones or fluctuating blood sugar and insulin levels often coincide with anxiety, phobias, trepidations, feelings of impending doom, dizziness, confusion, insecurity, frequent hunger pangs, and depression.

Mid-afternoon is often when the hypoglycemic will be overcome with fatigue or sleepiness. This author has found that corn often induces hypoglycemia. In Mexico, where corn is the main staple, what time do the people take their siesta? Yes, it's mid-afternoon. It is fascinating to see how different societies may counteract their hypoglycemia in different ways. In Britain, tea (caffeine) time is also 3-4 P.M. Corn sugar, also called dextrose, frequently causes a blood sugar reaction. If you are allergic to a food, you may react to anything that is derived from it. Sucrose (derived from cane or beets) is usually the worst. Organic maple syrup or rice syrup are often less allergenic than sucrose, dextrose or processed fructose — manufactured from dextrose — are. However, if your pancreas is weak — a rampant problem in the modern world — you are probably better off minimizing or eliminating simple sugars.

Allergies and hypoglycemia may be minimized by eating smaller, more frequent meals (as opposed to the daily, three, big ones). The old adage warns that we should "eat to live and not live to eat." *Small portions of food may be the way we were meant to eat.* Never forget, too, that hypoglycemia is nothing but a symptom of deeper problems — allergies, Candidiasis, etc.

Philpott recommends that *diabetics* have complete food allergy testing (with subsequent food elimination) as the allergenicity (or shock to the pancreas), not the amount of calories, is often the real key. Diabetics also need to be tested for allergy to the insulin they take. This is almost never done by diabetologists!

ADDICTION and ALLERGY

One of the hallmarks of allergy is *addiction* and its accompanying *withdrawal*. This is the allergy-addiction syndrome. Any food you crave, or like to eat often, is — or is likely to become — an allergy.

Many people don't want to admit their cravings and addictions. Some practitioners automatically denote a food as an allergy/addiction if it's eaten more than three times a week. In nature, there were no refrigerators or kitchen cupboards to allow habitual, eating patterns. Nor were most present-day foods, food combinations and amounts available. So your allergies will either be your favorite foods or, conversely, foods you know will make you ill. Foods that you "just don't care for" may be the best for you! They won't get you *high* as your allergenic foods do. Another clue that allergy may be the cause of a complaint is its *episodic* (come and go) nature. An infection, traumatized organ, or other possible cause should not manifest with an episodic nature as allergy does, due to the episodic exposure to the allergen.

Eating a food everyday without any "obvious" reaction is an example of the *masking effect*. That is, the worst symptoms are masked as the body attempts to adapt to the stress. Masking and allergy/addiction can also occur for chemicals, pollens etc. It can be shocking to find out *your favorite foods are your worst allergies*. But this is one of the causes of allergy. It's no coincidence that the most frequently eaten foods in our society are also the most common allergies. This includes wheat, corn, sugar, coffee, milk, peanuts, chocolate, eggs, oranges, tobacco, tomatoes, beef and yeast. One eats the foods one is allergic to everyday *precisely to avoid the effects of withdrawal*. Food addiction withdrawal can be as nightmarish as drug addiction withdrawal! One clinical ecologist recalls a woman patient begging him to kill her because she couldn't handle the withdrawal. Headache, fatigue, depression, arthritis and other symptoms are common. Food withdrawal lasts from 4-12 days, typically about 5 days. Chemical withdrawal can last up to 3 weeks. One can be masked for his/her own perfume (or cologne) which must also be eliminated. People often say, "Other people's perfumes bother me, but mine is O.K." If this person avoids her own perfume for a week and then uses it, she will get sick too! She was masked for it all along.

The person may even feel *better* after eating or breathing the allergen, in part because there is an adrenal rush. This phase has its ups and downs. But ingesting a small amount of an allergen or even a larger amount of a food that is only *slightly* allergenic to the body can actually cause a hyper reaction. Again the downside includes fatigue, depression, etc. Long before the term hyperactive was used, allergists described a "tension/fatigue" syndrome in children. The fatigue aspect referred to the fact that some children, after a hyper day, fell dead asleep at an early hour. Manic-depression too is likely the up and down reaction of allergy exposure and withdrawal. Some psychiatric journals have even published articles linking paranoia and schizophrenia to wheat and milk allergy. Most psychiatrists are, of course, not interested. We often say that 10% of psychiatrists recognize that wheat and milk can cause schizophrenia, and the other 90% eat wheat and milk!

Many people eat only 5-10 foods; going from one allergy-addiction to the next. We are an addicted society! The 24-hour convenience stores know about cravings and only stock foods that people will need a "fix" for. You won't find codfish there. We call these stores, "allergy/addiction headquarters."

One addiction begets another. The cigarette smoker and coffee drinker are probably allergic to these items, which *also induce hypoglycemia*. Former smokers are among the staunchest anti-smokers, because they were allergic to it all along! When eliminating an allergy/addiction, don't think of the rest of your life. During the initial withdrawal, think only of *five* days. At the end of the five days, you'll probably feel better than you have all your life. You'll want to stay on your optimum diet!

Let's return to caffeine and its connection to nicotine. The urge for a cigarette can be due to the caffeine just imbibed or to sugar or to a food in the *same food family* as tobacco (this includes tomato and potato) or to inhaling someone else's smoke. With appropriate action now, there doesn't have to be a miserable, lengthy withdrawal for the smoker as these other factors were causing some of the withdrawal. The worse the allergy — the worse the withdrawal. *And the more necessary to withdraw.*

ON ALCOHOLISM

Let's look more closely at alcoholism. In the 1950's, Theron Randolph, M.D. showed that alcoholism may not be addiction to alcohol as much as it is addiction to other food derivatives in the beverage.[54] This could be the source of the alcohol; e.g., wheat, rye (whiskey), potato (vodka), rice (sake), grapes (wine) or the sugar, yeast (beer), hops (beer), etc. that are added. In the early stages of alcoholism, there is usually a favorite beverage indicating allergy to a particular substance. The alcoholic thus needs complete allergy testing to avoid foods that are the cause of the "alcoholism." Eating such foods can cause a craving for the alcoholic beverage that contains it! Avoiding these foods may eliminate the miserable, lengthy withdrawal. At alcoholics' meetings, most members are eating cakes and drinking coffee (and smoking cigarettes). Thus the underlying allergies, hypoglycemia and Candidiasis are not being addressed. The last two disorders are likely involved if "any beverage will do" for the alcoholic.

Let's examine the *food family* concept more closely now. Related plant or animal foods may cross-react as they contain similar or identical proteins or other components. For example, grains (wheat, rye, barley, corn, oats, rice and millet) are grasses which may be similar to some airborne grass pollens. And all grains except rice and millet contain large amounts of the protein, gluten — which can cause gastrointestinal and brain symptoms in many.

With a long enough period of avoidance, *some* foods may again be tolerated on a *rotating basis*. This is because most allergies are said to be cyclical and not fixed. It is important after your allergy testing, that you do *not* start eating the same "safe" foods *every day* as these may become allergenic too.

Now you know that you likely need some form of food allergy testing. This can be done in many ways. We recommend against skin testing as the better allergists have always concluded that it's most accurate *only* for those who have skin allergies — a small percentage of allergic people. Newer blood tests include various types of RAST blood tests performed by physicians. Some "free" allergy tests include the following. Allergic foods are often undigested properly. If you can smell these foods in your urine or see them in your stool, you shouldn't eat them. We think the most accurate, the least expensive, and the quickest method can be Applied Kinesiology itself. (See Appendix B.)

CANDIDA ALBICANS & ITS HUMAN INTERACTION

We come now to the role of the yeast/fungus, Candida albicans, in chronic illness. Overgrowth of Candida albicans may be a cause of much chronic, degenerative, immunological and "emotional" illness. This includes allergy itself. We should note that Candida and other fungus and other germs are found in everyone's colon. It's also found in the air and on food. Only when overgrowth (or energy imbalance) occurs does illness ensue.

Let's start by listing possible symptoms of Candidiasis. Again allergies, other infectious agents and many other factors may cause some of these symptoms.

POSSIBLE SYMPTOMS OF CANDIDIASIS

Stool or breath with a moldy odor, female disorders — including vaginitis, PMS, endometriosis (the bacterium-like germ, chlamydia, may be at fault here), ovarian or uterine fibroids, sterility, infertility, male disorders — including prostatitis, allergies, coated tongue, bad breath, gas, bloating, pain, diarrhea, colitis, ileitis, constipation, ulcers, diaper rash, thrush, fungal nails and athlete's foot (other fungi are involved here, but it happens to people who have Candida problems), skin conditions, acne, psoriasis, heart: arrhythmias, mitral valve prolapse, low or high blood pressure, the author's discovery of "dyslexic heart," dyslexia, hyperactivity, headaches, migraines, fatigue, spaceyness, poor memory (often for names), poor balance, amnesia, M.S. (Multiple Sclerosis), addictions, especially sweets and yeast-containing foods, emotional, e.g. schizophrenia, earaches, especially in young children, asthma, sinusitis (if nutrition and diet change don't help with these two, Candida may be involved), bladder and kidney problems, immune deficiency, autoimmune disease, e.g. lupus, endocrine disorders, e.g., thyroid problems, problem pregnancy, problems with any moist, mucous membrane, vitreous floaters in the eyes, low or high blood sugar, Candida septicemia: Candida in the blood.

POSSIBLE CAUSES OF CANDIDIASIS

The following factors have led to the epidemic proportions of Candidiasis in modern, Western society: Antibiotics, birth control pills, cortisone drugs, excess sweets — sucrose is the worst, excess yeast containing foods, nutrient-poor food, artificial or junk food, starvation (Candidiasis is also rampant in starving Africa), foods with heated oils or other free radicals, allergies, sexual or intimate contact can pass this germ, endocrine disorders, toxicities, radiation, any immune system stress, fluoride toxicity, genetic predisposition, pregnancy, environmental mold exposure — either in your home (basement or bathroom) or local geographical area such as in humid areas, old age, and immune deficiency.

The leading culprit is thought to be *antibiotics*. Sometimes, just one episode of taking antibiotics (or the birth control pill) initiates a life-time of unfolding misery! Antibiotics will kill bacteria that may (or may not) be harming you; but they will also kill the friendly flora that live in our intestines. These helpful bacteria, such as the acidophilus strains, compete with any intestinal fungus and other germs and thus keep them from overgrowing. The acidophilus perform many other useful functions such as making vitamins and enzymes and their own antibiotics. But most antibiotic *medications* will kill off the acidophilus allowing the yeast a major victory. Now antibiotics have saved many lives in the last fifty years or so, but today they are terribly abused by Western physicians. Often a cold is really a viral infection (or even misdiagnosed allergies) and anti-bacterial medication is totally *inappropriate*. Our immune system, at its best, has a tough time against fungus. The extra help it gets from the friendly flora should not be obviated.

The *birth control pill* is composed of progesterone-like hormones that, as a side effect, alter the vaginal mucosa allowing Candida to overgrow. Yeast favor dark, moist or humid places whether it's in, or on the body, or in your basement. Increased progesterone is also released during pregnancy, accounting for the frequent, vaginal infections many women experience at that time.

Cortisone drugs weaken the immune system — they're used for this purpose in organ transplants — and also raise the blood sugar. Yeast also have receptors for similar type substances, so for all these reasons, this type of medication also favors yeast overgrowth. Mercury, dental filling — the so-called "silver amalgam" — has been found to be neurotoxic, immunotoxic and even antibiotic. Bacteria and fungus in the mouth can convert mercury into methylmercury which is even more toxic and antibiotic. The last fact means your acidophilus can again be killed.

Environmental mold exposure is an insidious and potentially overwhelming stress. Molds favor moist, dark places like air conditioning systems. To clean off molds, use borax, Zephiran or chlorine — maybe you can get someone who doesn't have allergies to do the job. Make sure your bedroom, bathroom, living room, etc. are not moldy. Certain geographical areas also favor large mold growth. These can include valleys, coasts and lake regions.

There is much in the modern diet that can lead to yeast overgrowth. The average diet is said to contain 100 times the sugar content that our grandparents ate at the turn of the century. Sucrose is the worst form of sugar and the favorite of the yeast. So eating foods with sucrose is feeding Candida's "sweet tooth." Any concentrated sweet can feed a yeast overgrowth. Fruits are replete with simple sugars. If you have a Candida problem, eat complex carbohydrates like grains, potatoes, sweet potatoes — and not simple carbohydrates — like fruits or sugar. Today's diet is also high in foods containing yeast and mold. You will need to avoid these foods to overcome a Candida problem *or mold allergy.*

FOODS CONTAINING YEAST AND MOLDS
These foods include the following. Cheese and other milk products, alcoholic beverages, anything aged, fermented, or

malted, vinegar or anything containing vinegar (mustard, ketchup, mayonnaise, salad dressings, pickles), soy sauce, tamari, dried fruits, mushrooms, MSG (Monosodium Glutamate), baker's yeast in baked goods — bacterial cultures and baking soda can be used as a substitute to make dough rise, and brewer's yeast. Brewer's yeast may be found in alcoholic beverages *and some vitamin supplements.* (Taking supplements with brewer's yeast was a major factor that nearly led to the author's untimely demise.) In the U.S., moldy, old fruits, that can't be sold, are often made into *fruit juice* and *baby food.* Avoid foods that pick up molds during their processing and storing. These can include peanuts and other nuts, grains, herbs, spices. Peanuts also contain the potent carcinogen, aflatoxin — a mold product. Anything that exposes much surface area can attract mold and other germs. This is why hamburger meat may cause a problem while steak may not. Similarly, any food left in the open for too long can pick up molds.

If you have the HAC (Hypoglycemia, Allergies, Candida) syndrome, avoid the fruity breakfasts which have unfortunately been favored in some recent best-sellers. You can eat for breakfast what you would eat at any other meal! Have some green vegetables with every meal, if possible.

SYMPTOMS OF CANDIDIASIS

Candidiasis can cause immunological, endocrinological, neurological, metabolic, and chronic, degenerative physical and emotional illness. A complete medical history and appropriate diagnostic tests can indicate if Candida is the culprit. Chances are that if a patient's complaints are varied, complex and not in a pattern that the physician may have memorized in medical school, Candidiasis should be considered.

Medical dogma holds that Candidiasis, *or other fungal disease* is limited to thrush (in the mouth), vaginitis, fungal nails, athlete's foot and Candida septicemia. The last is unchecked yeast growth in the blood in leukemia patients who have had their immune systems further compromised with radiation or chemotherapy.

Now as fungus favor moist, mucous membranes, it is easy to see how Candida can flourish anywhere in the gastrointestinal tract — from the mouth (thrush) to the anus (diaper rash). The lungs (asthma) and sinuses can also become "hangouts." Mucous membranes under the skin and in the ear passage ways may also be favored by yeast if the local ecology or immune system are compromised.

In its invasive form, Candida albicans grows mycelia — branch- or thread-like structures that can dig into human cells and extract nutrients. This can be one cause of a *permeable* gastrointestinal tract, which allows *undigested foods* to enter the blood and can therefore lead to allergies. Parasites, such as giardia and amoebas, can also cause this gastrointestinal permeability.

Candida can cause problems in the body *far* from where it may occur as an overgrowth. This is because its waste products may enter the blood and travel anywhere in the body. This author believes that Candida may be the cause of much hypoglycemia as follows. Low blood sugar may result from either a rapid growth of Candida or paradoxically from the *"die-off effect."* The greatest amount of toxins may be released during this period of die-off. Colonics may be recommended to flush out Candida before antifungals are given in order to reduce the number of organisms and thus the die-off. The die-off or *"Herxheimer Reaction"* for Candida may last for days or weeks. The greater the overgrowth is, the worse the die-off may be. Whatever symptoms existed, before anti-Candida treatment, may be exacerbated during the die-off.

This author has hypothesized that Candidiasis, can (directly or indirectly) be part of the cause of low or high blood sugar reactions. Thus the term, "HAC," (Hypoglycemia, Allergies, Candida.) Candida toxins from an overgrowth *or* a die-off may preferentially be absorbed by the pancreas. Our work also indicates that Candida toxins can cause some of the imbalances that you learned to correct in this book with applied kinesiology techniques.

ANTI-FUNGAL AGENTS

Natural substances used to combat Candida include iodine, Gentian Violet, garlic, Pau D'Arco, Australian Tea Tree Oil, cloves, echinecea, acidophilus — restoration of friendly intestinal bacteria, selenium, magnesium, and molybdenum. Selenium and magnesium are often crucial here. Consult an expert. Don't forget, the energy balancing techniques are crucial here.

Now that you know what allergies, blood sugar problems, and Candidiasis are all about — and how to counteract them — you are indeed more likely to enjoy a healthier and longer life!

APPENDIX B

MUSCLE BIOFEEDBACK TESTING or APPLIED KINESIOLOGY

It is not necessary to test for the imbalances corrected in this book. That's because doing the corrections — even if they were not needed — is not likely to cause an adverse reaction. These corrections are only harmless, energy balancings. However, there is a way to test for many of the imbalances revealed in this book. It is remarkably rapid, inexpensive and it can be quite accurate if you just practice it for a while. You can test for the lack of heart integration™ (dyslexic heart), the lack of brain hemisphere integration and all the other imbalances that we learned to correct in this book. This methodology is called Muscle Biofeedback Testing or Applied Kinesiology. We use these two terms interchangeably.

To test the body for imbalances, we need some *feedback system* to give us information on the body's current state and its reactions to external stimuli. Biofeedback[55] has become a familiar concept nowadays. Stress management and lie detectors — both *accepted* by mainstream medicine — make use of changes in skin cell electrical conductivity in response to something as "esoteric" as a thought or memory.

Small changes in muscle strength could also be used as a feedback system. Recall from chapter two that, in the 1960's, Goodheart discovered that individual muscles were energetically connected to corresponding acupuncture meridians. And these acupuncture meridians have been known for thousands of years to energize the body's organs. So there exists a feedback system of muscles to acupuncture meridians and from the meridians to the organs.

This is the *Muscle/Meridian/Organ* linkage. So by using muscle strength changes as feedback, the state of the related acupuncture meridian (as well as the muscle itself), could be immediately measured. Indirectly, the organ's energy status may be gauged by testing its related muscle, too. As the organ's energy state may not correlate with any pathological (disease) state, we should advise against misinterpreting muscle testing as "medical" in any way.

Though Applied Kinesiology was devised originally, by Goodheart, for testing muscle and spinal imbalances, it has been greatly expanded since then. The potential value for muscle testing and balancing in the health field is virtually limitless! It is used today by chiropractic physicians, medical physicians (including some allergists), dentists, nutritionists, psychologists, massage therapists, educators, vision therapists, and many others. Even in its simplest form, it can gauge imbalance and restore balance to muscles, meridians, spine, lymph, and circulatory systems. The key is that many imbalances can be *immediately* tested. Allergy testing is facilitated through Applied Kinesiology. Dentists can determine problems in teeth and psychologists can rapidly uncover and correct emotional stress.

Before we begin to perform our first muscle test, we need to list some factors that can affect its accuracy.

IDEAL MUSCLE BIOFEEDBACK TESTING CONDITIONS

Don't worry if you can't completely test in the following ideal circumstances. Just do the best you can.

Subject looks straight ahead during the tests. Don't hold breath, subject can breathe out during actual test. Don't strain or incorporate extraneous muscles or contort during the test. Do your best throughout the test, but *if* the muscle goes weak, let it go. Remove metal from body, especially electric watches, metal (jewelry) above the neck or that crosses the body's midline. Don't think negative thoughts which can cause weak responses, keep the mind "blank." Wear loose-fitting, cotton clothes, lighter colors are best. Be in natural lighting. Avoid extraneous sounds. Don't test if subject is hungry or thirsty.

The preamble below can correct some *"switching"* that might be created by less-than-ideal conditions. But be aware that being switched doesn't just mean your testing may be somewhat inaccurate. It also means your energy and health are affected. All these factors can potentially cause what kinesiologists call "switching" or *neurological disorganization*. That is, they can create imbalances in the body's circuits that can cause a muscle response opposite to the "unswitched" or true response. There is a temporary, unswitching preamble that can help ensure accuracy. Using muscle biofeedback testing, without taking these precautions, may be inaccurate.

UNSWITCHING PREAMBLE FOR SUBJECT

(1) Simultaneously rub the navel and the two points above the upper lip and below the lower lip as in Figure 51.

(2) Simultaneously rub the navel and the two K27 points. See Figure 51. The K (or kidney) 27 points are (acupuncture meridian) points under the collar bone, adjacent to the sternum. (The latter is the bone running down the center, to which the ribs attach.)

(3) Rub the navel and the coccyx (tailbone, not shown) which is just above the anus.

Rub each set of two-hand corrections for 10 seconds. These three corrections temporarily correct top-bottom, left-right, and front-back switching, respectively. These three dimensions are also known as Pitch, Roll and Yaw. They relate to the body knowing where it is in three dimensional space.

Now we're ready. Here we will refer to Figures 52 and 53. Have the subject extend his/her arm straight out to the side and the testor will stand in front and off-center a bit. Don't be directly in front. Stabilize the opposite shoulder with your non-testing hand as shown. This helps prevent contortion; some will want to employ muscles other than the one being tested.

Figure 51.

Unswitching Points. Rub these points while holding the navel. Also add the coccyx point (not shown).

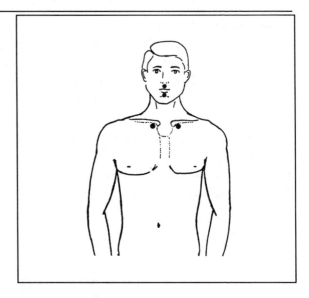

MUSCLE TESTING RULES

1. Ask if any injuries are present before you start.

2. Subject will say "stop" if pain should arise.

3. Testor will place his/her fingers, or hand, flat on top of the arm just below the wrist. Do not grip, or squeeze, the arm.

4. Testor will say "hold" just before pressing down towards the floor.

5. Testor may show the range of motion to the subject first. That is, without the subject resisting, take the subject's arm and push it down several inches.

6. Now the subject will hold the arm up as shown in Figures 52 and 53, and attempt to lock out the muscle and prevent the arm from moving towards the floor as the testor gently begins pushing the arm in this direction.

7. Testor builds up pressure *very slowly. During the first second of pressure build-up, hardly any force is used.* This is crucial to allow the subject to actually *feel* what is occurring!

8. Testor pushes for about 2 seconds.

9. With steady pressure, push down the arm only until testor is sure of response. If weak, there's no need to drag the arm down more

Figure 52.

Muscle Testing
Procedure.
See also Figure 53.

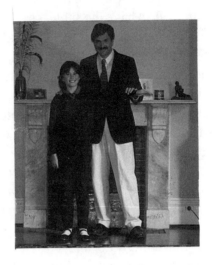

Figure 53.

Muscle testing
procedure you will start
using today!

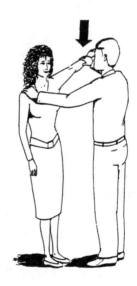

than 6 inches.

When learning, the most common mistake is to push *too hard, too soon*. A small percentage of people push *too lightly* and don't seem to want to have a weak response show up on their friend. One test for accuracy is to have the subject say a true statement such as "My name is (his/her actual name.)" Quickly muscle test. It should be strong. If the subject says "My name is (a name not his/her own)," s/he should muscle test weak. This assumes you have taken care of switching.

When you're proficient at muscle biofeedback testing, you can check for two additional imbalances. Test for dehydration by first testing to see if you have a strong muscle. This is called testing in *the clear*, as you're not testing anything but the muscle itself. It's also called finding a *"strong indicator muscle."* The dehydration test is to simply (gently) pull some hair on the subject's head while testing the strong indicator muscle. If the muscle tests weak, provide some pure water and retest in a few seconds. It should now be strong! We're mostly water and dehydration readily weakens (and switches) the body. (Shaky muscles can also result.) Next we will refer to Figure 54 for testing blood sugar energy imbalance.

"BLOOD SUGAR ENERGY TEST"

1. Place the thumb one inch above the navel and
2. Simultaneously place the middle and pointer fingers (which are touching each other at the tips) at the point one inch to the subject's left (of the thumb).
3. Test the strong indicator muscle now.
4. If weak, recommend the subject eat some safe food or perform the energy balance known as the "blood sugar energy balance" as described on page 87.

The energy imbalances created by dehydration and faulty blood sugar need to be tested and corrected for accurate muscle biofeedback testing.

Take the time to perfect your "feel" or feedback on the results of your muscle tests. Vary your pressure with the strength of the subject. Use a greater force (but still come in slowly) for the Schwartzeneggers and a much lesser force for a five year old girl. Remember this is *not* a contest of wills or muscles. It is a test to see if a muscle *locks* in regard to a specific challenge at the time of the

Figure 54.

Blood sugar energy
test points.

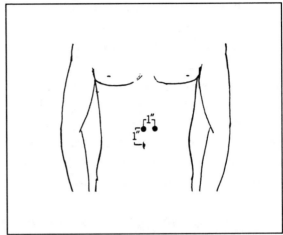

test. The fascinating thing is that a weak response is only 10%, or
so, less strong than the "strong" response. This is why this subtle
response monitoring wasn't observed until recently.

After some preliminary testing, you should know whether a
muscle is strong or not. (This is the whole ball game here.) We're
now ready to test for environmental sensitivities.

Our testing involves "energy" testing only. If a substance is placed
on the body, muscle biofeedback testing can be utilized with great
accuracy! This is hypothesized to work as follows. Every substance
in the Universe has its own characteristic electromagnetic field; and
the acupuncture meridians (near the skin) are also electromagnetic
in nature. An allergen would thus have a field that would be
disharmonious to the body's meridian energies. This weakens the
meridian which in turn weakens our muscles by that almost imper-
ceptible 10%.

TESTING FOR SENSITIVITIES

1. Hold the food over each of the first five regions or points.
2. Simultaneously, muscle test with the food held at each point or
region.
We use the *TESTING SCHEME* shown in Figure 55.

We test here for energy imbalances or sensitivities, not medical
allergies. Region 1 involves the pancreas/spleen. Region 2 is the

liver. Point 3 is the "triple warmer alarm point" of acupuncture theory, an inch below the navel. (This point measures endocrine imbalance.) Region 4 is the thymus.

If you get a weak muscle test result at even one place, stop. You have uncovered an energy sensitivity. And never press the substance into the body, rather gently hold against the body.

This scheme is a guide that should be changed if the circumstances warrant it. For example, if a physician suspects a food is causing arthritis at the knee, he can place the food *there* and test! (Over half of a person's sensitivities seem to involve liver or pancreas energy imbalance.) These results may not show up on traditional, medical allergy testing. Most of these tests are known to be *inaccurate* for foods. This is why many allergists leave their patients to suffer and *completely ignore food allergies* and just deal with pollen allergies — even though these patients will always have food allergies that are affecting them more than the pollen allergies are!! The Muscle Biofeedback Testing can pick up *95%* of a person's "sensitivities."

Test a mono (or single item) food, not combo foods. Don't leave foods lying on the body for more than 10 seconds as the body's energies may "adapt" to the stress. This type of testing offers possibilities that all other testing can't. You can test fluorescents,

Figure 55.

Sensitivity testing
scheme.

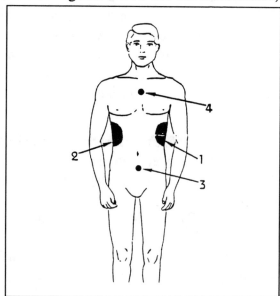

T.V.'s, sounds, colors etc. You can test things by looking at them or by being under or near them; as long as your senses pick it up. Getting back to food, if an apple gives a weak response, you can separately test the skin, seeds, and meat. If the skin muscle-tests weak, it may be due to mold or pesticide. Try an organic apple!

To accurately test for vitamin sensitivities, we devised an additional step. Simply break off the tiniest piece and use the same points of Figure 55 for testing!

Always remember, the most accurate test is reality itself. But Muscle Biofeedback Testing, when used optimally, can be quick, inexpensive, non-symptom-provoking and accurate.

Let's see how we can test for the need to perform the Rochlitz Heart Integration™ Exercises.

HEART INTEGRATION™ TESTING SCHEME
1. Draw a large "X" on a blank piece of paper.
2. Test your strong indicator muscle. Make sure it locks (strong.)
3. Place the subjects hand over his heart. This should test strong.
4. Next, with the hand still over the heart, the subject views the "X." Hold up the "X" at the subject's eye level and about a foot away.
5. Simultaneously, muscle test now. If the muscle goes weak, the non-medical condition of "dyslexic heart" exists.

Someone with a heart disease may well test strong, signaling an integrated heart. And someone with a perfect heart may test weak— the hemispheres, at the moment, are not integrated. So this does not relate to any medical conditions.

Now we're ready to go to a simple "hands on" testing for the lack of brain hemisphere integration.

TESTING FOR BRAIN HEMISPHERE INTEGRATION
1. Draw a large "X" on a blank piece of paper.
2. Make sure you have a strong indicator muscle.
3. Hold up the "X" directly (about 10 inches) in front of the subject at their eye level.

4. Simultaneously, muscle test again — this is the actual test. If weak, you have uncovered a lack of brain integration. Don't diagnose dyslexia, because that's just a name and you will momentarily make the correction anyway.

TESTING FOR HAND or FOOT GAIT REFLEXES

Here the test for either the hand or foot gait points is to merely touch each point while muscle testing.

Figure 56.

Foot gait reflex points.

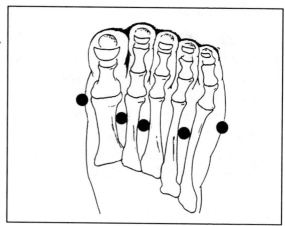

Figure 57.

Hand gait reflex points.

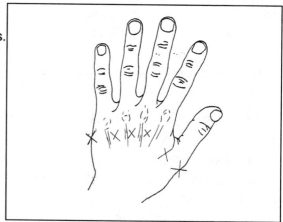

APPENDIX C — RESOURCES

Human Ecology Balancing Sciences (H.E.B.S.), Inc.
P.O. Box 737 Mahopac, N.Y. 10541 U.S.A.
Phone: (914) 228-4162   Fax: (914) 228-4615

You can use the methods of this book and more advanced ones to achieve wellness or to attain certification status — should you wish to make a career or vocation of these methods. You may write to us for the name of the nearest certified H.E.B.S. instructors who can perform educational, research and non-medical energy testing and balancing and can teach the H.E.B.S. classes. It's well worth traveling large distances to see one of our certified graduates! *Enclose a stamped, self-addressed envelope.*

This offers a more detailed view of the methods of this book. The author teaches the Basic and Advanced H.E.B.S. seminars around the world. You may also contact us about sponsoring these seminars and we will send you information on the prerequisites. If you are unaware of the cause of your complaints, seeing a physician first is wise. However, we have observed that it's a good idea not to put all your hopes and finances in one "basket." When someone can help you, you'll usually feel it in one visit! We devised the Human Ecology Balancing Sciences system to offer instruction and non-medical sessions covering the realms of ecology, nutrition, integration exercises and kinesiology.

While we strongly recommend only our own certified Instructor-Practitioners for the very best results, you can check your yellow pages under chiropractic, naturopathic (and maybe even osteopathic and medical) physicians. See who lists *Applied Kinesiology* in their listing.

In Canada, contact Certified H.E.B.S. Instructor-Practitioner, Irene Yaychuk, Ph.D. 48 Huron St. Brantford, ONT N3S 2J6 CANADA (519) 759-3524

German-speaking people can contact Certified H.E.B.S. Instructor-Practitioner, Timothy Kaufmann at Paul Ehrlich Str. 22 D-5270 Gummersbach 1 GERMANY

APPENDIX D

BIBLIOGRAPHY

1. Rochlitz, Steven. "Heart and Brain Integration: A New Unified Approach." *International Journal of Touch For Health*; 1986:24-26.
2. Cantin, Marc and Genest, Jacques. "The Heart as an Endocrine Gland." *Scientific American.* 254:2 76-81
3. "Heart Peptide Goes to the Head." *Science News.* 131:68.
4. Rochlitz, Steven. *Allergies and Candida: with the Physicist's Rapid Soluiton 1988 (1st Ed.), 1991 (3rd Ed.)* New York: Human Ecology Balancing Sciences, Inc.
5. Rochlitz, Steven. See references 1 and 4.
6. Ibid
7. "New Non-Invasive Test For Dyslexia." *The Human Ecology Balancing Scientist* Vol. I, #4
8. "Proof Of Increased Stretch After The Rochlitz Heart Integration." *The Human Ecology And Energy Balancing Scientist* Vol 3 #3.
9. *"Meta-Integration Breakthrough Announced."* The Human Ecology Balancing *Scientist* Vol. I, #1
10. Ibid.
11. Rowe, Albert H. and Albert Jr. *Food Allergy, Its Manifestations And Control And The Elimination Diets: A Compendium.* C.C. Thomas, 1972.
12. J. Karjalainen et al. "A Bovine Peptide as a Possible Trigger of Insulin Dependent Diabetes Mellitus." *New England Journal of Medicine*; 1992, 327: 302-7.
13. "Dr. Spock Warns on Cow's Milk." *Facts on File.* 1992 p. 794
14. Goodheart, Robert and Shils, Maurice. *Modern Nutrition In Health And Disease: Dietotherapy. 5th Ed.* Philadelphia: Lea & Febiger 1976.
15. Livingston-Wheeler, Virginia and Addeo, Edmund. *The Conquest Of Cancer: Vaccines And Diet.* New York: Franklin Watts, 1984.
16. Formaldehyde and Other Toxins Related to Brain Dysfunction; *The Human Ecology Balancing Scientist.* Vol. II. No. 1.
17. "More On Aspartame As Brain Killer" *The Human Ecology Balancing Scientist* Vol. 2, No.2 Sept. 1988.
18. Kirschmann, John D. *Nutrition Alamanac.* New York: Mcgraw Hill, 1984
19. "Aspirin: to prevent heart attacks?" *Consumer Reports.* Oct. 1988; p 616-8.
20. "New Form Of Vitamin C Helps Some To Take Vitamin C Without Bladder Frequency Symptoms" *The Human Ecology & Energy Balancing Scientist.* Vol 3 #4
21. Schaumberg, Herbert et al."Sensory Neuropathy from Pyridoxine Abuse." *The New England Journal of Medicine*; 1983, 309:445-7.
22. "Drilling for Danger." *Newsweek,* Oct. 15, 1990; p. 80.
23. Deng, Han-Xiang, et al. "ALS and Structural Defects in Cu, Zn Superoxide Dismutase." *Science.* 261:1047-1050.
24. Dry, J. and Pradalier, A. "Histamine Antagonists." *Antihormones,* Agarwal,

ED. Elsevier: North Holland Biomedical Press, 1979.

25. Philpott, William et al.: "The Role of Addiction in the Mental Disease Process," *The Journal Of Applied Nutrition*, 1980, 32:20-36.

26. Freed, D. "Allergens as Poisons: Airborne and Food-Borne Toxins." *Clinical Ecology*. 1986; 4:1 21-25.

27. *Physician's Desk Reference*, 42nd Ed. Medical Economics, 1988.

28. Lust, John. *The Herb Book*. New York: Bantam Books, 1980.

29. Thie, John F. *Touch For Health*, Marina Del Rey: De Vorss & Co., 1979.

30. Walther, David. *Applied Kinesiology: Vol I. Basic Procedures And Muscle Testing*. Pueblo: Systems DC, 1981.

31. Rochlitz, Steven. *Allergies and Candida*.

32. "More On Aspartame As Brain Killer" *The Human Ecology Balancing Scientist* Vol. 2, No.2. Sept. 1988.

33. *Wholemind*, August 1988.

34. "New Study On The Dangers Of Aspartame" *The Human Ecology Balancing Scientist* Vol. 2, No. 4 March 1989.

35. *Journal Of Applied Nutrition*. Vol. 40, No. 2.

36. "Verification Of Tenet Of Rochlitz Aldehyde Dyslexia Hypothesis" *The Human Ecology Balancing Scientist* Vol. 2, No. 3. Jan. 1989.

37. Karl, Peter. "Acetaldehyde Production And Transfer By The Perfused Placental Cotyledon." *Science*, Oct. 14. 1988.

38. Papaioannou, R., Pfeiffer, C. "Sulfite Sensitivity—Unrecognized Threat: Is Molybdenum the Cause?" *Journal of Orthomolecular Psychiatry*; 1984, 13:105-110.

39. See Reference 16.

40. "Exercise Helps CFS." *The Human Ecology & Energy Balancing Scientist* 4:2

41. "TV Causes Depression." *The Human Ecology&Energy Balancing Scientist*.4:3

42. Rochlitz, Steven. *Allergies and Candida:*

43. "Fibromyositis" *The Human Ecology And Energy Balancing Scientist Vol 6 #2*

44. *Science*. Nov. 8, 1991. P. 797.

45. "Maestro & Giving Blood" *Human Ecology & Energy Balancing Scientist* 3:1

46. After Heart Integration, Physician Wonders—Is This Two Different People? *The Human Ecology And Energy Balancing Scientist* Vol 3 #3

47. "Rochlitz Heart Integration Warms Up Cold Hand." *The Human Ecology And Energy Balancing Scientist* Vol 4 #1

48. "Blood Pressure Normalized With Rochlitz Heart Integration." *The Human Ecology Balancing Scientist* Vol 1 #4.

49. Ibid

50. Ibid

51. Mackarness, Richard. *Eating Dangerously: The Hazards Of Hidden Allergy*. New York: Harcourt, Brace, Jovanovich, 1976.

52. Philpott, William and Kalita, Dwight. *Brain Allergies: The Psychonutrient Connection*. New Canaan: Keats, 1980

53. Philpott, William and Kalita, Dwight. *Victory Over Diabetes: A Bio-ecologic Triumph*. New Canaan: Keats, 1983.

54. Randolph, Theron and Moss, Ralph. *An Alternative Approach To Allergies*. New York: Bantam Books, 1982.

55. Brown, Barbara. *NEW MIND, NEW BODY*. New York: Harper and Row, 1974.

Index

acetaldehyde, 33, 73 - 75
acetylcholine, 74
acidophilus, 120 - 121
acupuncture meridians, 13, 15 - 16, 125 - 126, 131
addiction, 29 - 30, 32, 53, 56, 78 - 79, 82, 115 - 119
adrenal, 29, 30, 37, 51, 78, 79, 114, 115, 117
aflatoxin, 122
alcohol, 33, 38, 55, 61, 79
alcoholism, 115, 118, 122
allergy, 12, 22, 29 - 32, 35 - 37, 112 - 116, 118 - 124
allergy/addiction, 30, 32, 36, 50, 57
ALS, 51
Alzheimer's Disease, 34, 68, 73, 76
amoebas, 123
anti-fungal agents, 123
anti-oxidants, 41 - 42, 46 - 48, 50 - 51
antibiotics, 120 - 121
appestat, 53
Applied Kinesiology, 1, 12, 15, 73, 81 - 83, 89 - 91, 119, 126
arm jogging, 15
arrhythmias (cardiac), 12 - 13, 108, 109, 113, 119
arthritis, 12, 35, 51, 78, 113, 116, 132
aspartame, 35, 38, 74
aspirin, 45 - 46, 51
banana, 60 - 61
beans, 60 - 61
beef, 44, 54
beta carotene, 47
bioflavonoids, 41 - 42, 46, 48 - 49
blood pressure, 13 - 14, 22, 27, 31, 33, 60 - 63, 66 - 67, 108, 110, 113
blood sugar energy correction, 87
blood sugar energy test, 130
brain hemisphere, 21, 68 - 71, 73 - 75
brain integration exercise, 71, 73, 84
brain integration test, 133
bruising, 13, 22, 108

caffeine, 22, 29 - 31, 38, 44, 54, 78 - 79, 81, 115, 117
calcium, 31, 43, 52, 79 - 80
cancer, 11, 37, 114
Candida, 36, 55, 62, 75, 79 - 81, 112 - 113, 115, 119 - 123
car sickness, 69
cardiovascular nutrients, 40
carnitine, 41, 43
cataracts, 50
cats, 98
chocolate, 29
cholesterol, 32 - 33, 42 - 43
cigarette, 117
citrus, 32, 35, 48 - 49, 60 - 61
Coenzyme Q_{10}, 41, 44
coffee, 29, 117 - 118
cola, 29
cold hands and feet, 22, 108, 110
conductor (music), 15 - 16
corn, 36, 115 - 116, 118
corpus callosum, 69 - 70, 73 - 74, 76
cortisone, 121
counting, 16 - 18, 27, 57, 71, 83
cranial correction, 77, 80, 81, 99, 111
cross-lateralness, 69
cross-crawl, 15, 19, 24, 63, 71 - 73, 84
cysteine, 46, 50
Cytomegalovirus, 79
dairy (cheese, milk), 31 - 33, 35, 38, 44, 52, 54 - 56, 60, 67, 74, 79, 81, 90, 98, 112 - 113, 116, 121
decaffeinated coffee, 30 - 31
depression, 59, 113 - 117
diabetes, 114
Die-off reaction, 123
disordered methionine, 54
diuresis, 54
dumping syndrome, 77, 81
dyslexia, 21, 68, 72 - 75, 134
dyslexic heart, 21, 133
ears — switching on, 86

elderly, 44, 69 - 71
endorphin, 55 - 56
environmental mold, 121
epilepsy, 43
Epstein-Barr Virus, 77, 79, 82 - 83
Eskimo, 32, 43
exercise, 79, 89 - 90, 92, 96
exorphins, 55
fatigue, 12 - 13, 27, 30, 77 - 83, 85, 87, 90, 92, 94, 106, 112, 114 - 117, 119
fatigue: distinguishing causes list, 82
fats, 43, 114
fermented foods, 32, 60 - 61
fibromyalgia (fibromyositis), 82
fish, 36 - 38, 41, 43, 47, 50, 52
fluorescent lights, 112, 132
food combining, 37
food family, 118
formaldehyde, 51, 73 - 76
free radical, 33-34, 41, 46, 47, 50, 120
gait reflexes, 85, 94, 95, 105, 106, 134
gall bladder, 37
garlic, 62, 123
Giardia, 123
ginger, 62
giving blood (& Maestro), 108
glutathione, 46, 50
gluten, 55, 114, 118
gout, 59
HAC (Syndrome), 123
hand gaits, 95, 106
headaches, 116, 119
heart attack, 43
heart hemispheres, 16, 21
heart integration™, 16, 18, 23, 25, 70 - 71, 109 - 111
Heart Integration Exercise™, 19, 63, 97, 99, 101, 108 - 109, 111
Heart Integration™ Test, 133
Herpes, 79
Herxheimer Reaction, 123
histamine, 31, 53 - 54, 78

histidine, 52
homogenized (milk), 31
homolateral (crawl), 19, 72
humming, 16 - 17, 19, 27, 63, 65, 71, 73, 83 - 84
hydrochloric acid, 44
hyperactivity, 117
hypoglycemia, 30, 54, 76, 78 - 80, 82, 114 - 115, 117 - 118, 122 - 123
hypothalamus, 53 - 54, 77 - 78
immune system, 49 - 50, 119 - 122
immunodeficiency, 114
insulin, 115
interferon, 46
kidney, 14, 16, 26, 36 - 37, 43, 50, 54, 59 - 60, 119
labor time, 108, 111
lactose, 31
lecithin, 41, 43
left brain, 69 - 70
leg abduction test, 23, 26
lipid peroxides, 50
liver, 15, 29, 48 - 49, 55, 76
longevity, 11, 13, 16, 18, 21, 26 - 29, 31, 33, 34, 36, 38, 48, 51 - 52, 112, 124
lupus, 51, 114, 120
multiple sclerosis (M.S.), 13, 15, 22, 81, 97 - 101, 103, 106 - 107
Maestro Exercise™, 16 - 17, 21, 27, 65, 83, 100, 101, 108, 111
magnesium, 41, 43, 45, 52, 77, 79 - 80, 124
margarine, 38
masking effect, 116
Max EPA® fish oil, 41, 43, 52
meat, 33 - 34, 37 - 38, 43, 56, 122
mercury (& amalgam), 50, 114, 121
Meta-Maestro™, 27, 28, 65
methanol, 74
microwaved food, 33 - 35, 38, 112
Mitral Valve Prolapse, 119
mold, 33, 78 - 80, 82

ASK YOUR BOOK STORE OR LIBRARY TO ORDER ADDITIONAL COPIES OF THIS BOOK FOR YOU THROUGH THEIR DISTRIBUTORS or CONTACT US

TO LEARN MORE ABOUT OUR SEMINARS & OTHER PUBLICATIONS:

Please contact: Human Ecology Balancing Sciences, Inc.
P. O. Box 737
Mahopac, N.Y. 10541 USA Phone: (914) 228-4162 Fax: (914) 228-4615
The Human Ecology Balancing Sciences [HEBS] Seminars are the world's only wellness seminars covering human ecology, nutrition, muscle biofeedback testing and heart/brain/meridian integration exercises.™ Learning, vision correction, and other topics are also covered. The H.E.B.S. seminars provide the best methods for optimum physical and mental functioning. They're also great for athletes and business executives who need that extra edge. *Please enclose an SASE —self-addressed, stamped envelope. Thanks!*

ALLERGIES & CANDIDA: WITH THE PHYSICIST'S RAPID SOLUTION, Third Edition

By Prof. STEVEN ROCHLITZ

 Simply put, this is the most complete and essential health book you can buy!

272 pages, 44 illustrations, ISBN 0-945262-21-3 (soft) ISBN 0-945262-20-5 (Hard)
Softcover: $19.95 or *Limited, Deluxe, Autographed Hardcover:* $23.95
Published by Human Ecology Balancing Sciences, Inc. (H.E.B.S., Inc.)
P.O. Box 737 Mahopac, N.Y. 10541 USA, Phone: (914) 228-4162 Fax: (914) 228-4615
SHIPPING: $3.75 in the U.S. (U.P.S. — give your street address, $1.00 per additional book. Overseas: $8.50 for air mail. Surface (including Canada): $2.00
New Yorkers : add sales tax.

SEE ORDER FORM TWO PAGES DOWN.

Retail stores: Contact your distributor or wholesaler or call or write us for your discount schedule.

Coming in 1994...*The VIDEO* of All The Corrections In This *Book!*

WHY DO MUSIC CONDUCTORS LIVE INTO THEIR _90'S?_

The Simple, Revolutionary Discovery That Can Make You Live Longer, Increase Your Stamina & Stretch, And Normalize Your Blood Pressure In Minutes

By Prof. STEVEN ROCHLITZ

Price: $12.95   140 pages, 57 Illustrations. ISBN: 0-945262-42-6
Shipping: _USA_: $2.00 for 4th class mail (non-insured), _or_ $4.00 for U.P.S. (insured) in the continental USA (to street address.)
To Canada & Overseas: Surface mail (non-insured): $2.00; or Air mail: $7.00 Add $1.00 per additional book. Insurance is additional except for UPS to USA.
Published by Human Ecology Balancing Sciences, Inc. (HEBS, Inc.)
P.O. Box 737 Mahopac, N.Y. 10541 USA Phone: (914) 228-4162 Fax: (914) 228-4615

THE REFERENCE, WALL CHART

For only $29.95, you can have a _four-color, 2 ft. by 3 ft., double-side-laminated,_ reference, wall chart depicting _all_ the corrections and tests of this book _plus_ others not found here and the _first_ reference telling you which corrections to make for which complaints! Contains 35 photos and illustrations and text for the tests & corrections. Shipping: $4.00 everywhere. $8.50-air mail to overseas.

THE ADVANCED HUMAN ECOLOGY AND ENERGY BALANCING MANUAL

In 1985, Rochlitz extrapolated the concept of integration exercises beyond the brain and heart to include all the meridian/organ systems. These Rochlitz Meridian Integration™ Exercises utilize the applied kinesiology muscle for all the appropriate muscle/meridian/organ systems in analogous cross-crawl fashion. This advanced manual continues where _Allergies and Candida: with the Physicist's Rapid Solution_ leaves off. Advanced balancing techniques include: How to balance the body's energies for energy imbalance from allergies and Candida imbalance. Includes the body points for vitamins, minerals, digestants and amino acids for rapid kinesiological testing and balancing.
ISBN: 0-945262-40-X 100 pages, 8.5" by 11" With 28 illustrations and leatherette cover; spiral bound so it can be opened flat for easy reference. Price: $59.95 plus $4.00 shipping. Overseas air mail: $8.00.

Quantity Discounts On All Books & Tapes
10-19 ⇒30% off
20-39⇒40% off
40 or more ⇒50% off
U.P.S. shipping: $0.50 per book—**At least 10 books.**
Overseas (Surface)—$1.00 per book.

SUBSCRIBE TO OUR QUARTERLY NEWSLETTER

THE HUMAN ECOLOGY & ENERGY BALANCING SCIENTIST
Editor-in-Chief: Prof. Steven Rochlitz

The world's only quarterly newsletter with regular updates and breakthroughs in Human Ecology, Nutrition, Kinesiology and Heart/Brain/Meridian Integration Exercises.™ And the way to find out about future publications, special sales and our classes.

ISSN: 1045-2729. Shipped air mail. [Sample, or back, issues, $3.00 each.]

1 Year (4 issues)	2 Years (8 issues)
$14.95—U.S.	$27.95—U.S.
$15.95—Canada	$29.95—Canada
$17.95—Overseas	$33.95—Overseas

HEALING/RELAXATION TAPE FOR OVERCOMING ALLERGIES (Side A) & *CANDIDA* (Side B).
Narrated by Prof. Steven Rochlitz

60-minute, audio cassette tape — $9.95. Surface shipping: $2.00, except overseas: $3.00. Air mail, overseas: $4.50.

ABOUT THE AUTHOR

.. Steven Rochlitz is perhaps the world's only .iysicist/Nutritionist/Kinesiologist. He has been a member of the American Institute of Physics, the American Association of Physicists in Medicine, the American Association for the Advancement of Science, the New York Academy of Science, and the International Acedemy of Nutrition and Preventive Medicine. His degrees (from the City College of New York and the State University of New York at Stony Brook) are all in Physics. During his five years in graduate Physics, Rochlitz received the prestigious National Science Foundation Graduate Research Fellowship for doctoral research in astrophysics and mathematical biology. He taught both graduate and undergraduate Physics at two Universities by the age of 23.

In the early 1980's, he became an expert in the new science of Applied Kinesiology. Rochlitz went on to teach his methods, to both laymen and physicians, around the world. Rochlitz' discoveries have led to his inclusion in *Who's Who in Science & Engineering* and to radio and T.V. appearances around the world. He has published tapes and articles in health and medical journals and is also Editor-in-Chief of *The Human Ecology & Energy Balancing Scientist.* He is the creator of Heart Integration,™ Meridian Integration,™ and Meta-Integration™ Exercises, and the Candida Balance.™ Rochlitz' first book, *Allergies and Candida: with the Physicsit's Rapid Solution* has become a best-seller in several languages. This is his third health/self-help book.